What Women Really Want in Bed

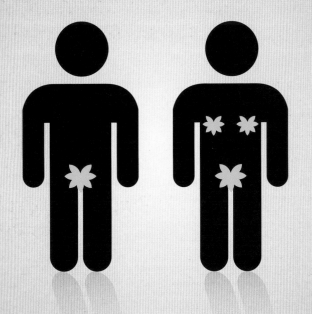

What Women Really Want in Bed

The Surprising Secrets Women Wish Men Knew About Sex

Cynthia W. Gentry
and **Dana Fredsti**

QUIVER

Text © 2010 Cynthia W. Gentry and Dana Fredsti

First published in the USA in 2010 by
Quiver, a member of
Quayside Publishing Group
100 Cummings Center
Suite 406-L
Beverly, MA 01915-6101
www.quiverbooks.com

14 13 12 11 10   1 2 3 4 5

ISBN-13: 978-1-59233-339-4
ISBN-10: 1-59233-339-7

Library of Congress Cataloging-in-Publication Data available

Cover and book design by Traffic
Book layout: Rachel Fitzgibbon

Printed and bound in Singapore

Dedications

To Nima, as always.

To Dave, who never stops trying to answer this question.

Contents

Chapter 1: What *Do* Women Really Want in Bed?   **8**
How to Find Out What *Your* Woman Wants in Bed   13

Chapter 2: Fabulous Foreplay   **14**
What Women Wish Men Knew about Foreplay   16
What Kind of Foreplay Gets Women the Hottest?   22
Her Body Is a Wonderland: Her Erogenous Zones   27
Foreplay: What Not to Do   28
Good Things Come to Those Who Wait   31

Chapter 3: Hands On   **32**
What Women Wish Men Knew about Using Their Hands   34
Push My Buttons (The Right Ways)   40
Push My Buttons (The Wrong Ways)   44
Top Hand Techniques   47
Let Your Fingers Do the Talking   51

Chapter 4: Oral Sex: The Good, the Bad, and the Ugly   **54**
What Women Wish Men Knew About Oral Sex   56
The Biggest Mistake Men Make During Oral Sex   64
Finding the Best Rhythm and Pressure   66
The Sexiest Thing to Do with Your Mouth   69
Her Geography of Desire   73
What Women Wish Men Knew about Fellatio   75

Chapter 5: The Main Event   **80**
What Women Wish Men Knew about the "The Act"   82
Does Size Matter?   87
Location, Location, Location   90
Can We (Dirty) Talk?   94
Favorite Positions   96
What's the Frequency?   102
Crashing & Burning: A How-To Guide   106
Parting Words   109

Chapter 6: All about Orgasms   **110**
In Search of the Big O   112
Surefire Orgasm Techniques   115
Faking It   118
The Truth about Multiple Orgasms   122

Chapter 7: The Afterglow   **124**
What Women Wish Men Knew about the Afterglow   126
Ending a Bang with a Whimper: The Biggest After-Sex Turnoffs   134
How to Be Rude in Four Easy Steps   139
The Bottom Line   141

Chapter 8: Flights of Fantasy   **142**
What Women Wish Men Knew about Their Sexual Fantasies   144
What is She Fantasizing About?   150
Let the Games Begin   154
Not Her Game   156
Toy Time   158
The Pornography Question   159
Tie Me Up, Tie Me Down: BDSM   163
Will You Share her Wilder Side?   166

Appendix: How to Get A Woman *into* Bed: Secrets of Seduction   **168**
What Women Wish Men Knew about Seduction   170
What's the First Thing Women Notice about a Guy?   179
What Part of Your Body Does She Find the Sexiest?   184
The Brass Tacks of Seduction   188
Game Killers   190
How Soon Is Too Soon (or Not Soon Enough)?   191
You Go First. No, YOU Go First!   193
How to Keep Things Going   197

Acknowledgments   200
About the Authors   202
Index   204

Chapter 1

What *Do* Women Really Want in Bed?

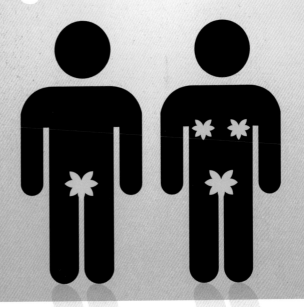

Are you, like Freud, puzzled by women and their sexual desires? Do you wonder, for example, whether your girlfriend or wife really likes giving—and getting—oral sex? Does she fantasize when making love to you? What does she really need to have an orgasm? What kinds of fantasies is she having? All things you might wonder about, but never feel comfortable enough to ask your gal. So we asked for you. And boy, did we get answers.

"The great question...which I have not yet been able to answer, despite my thirty years of research 'What does a woman want?' "

Sigmund Freud, the father of psychoanalysis

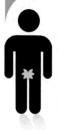

But before we delve into them, some background. In 2005, one of your coauthors, Cynthia Gentry, decided that she'd had enough of so-called experts telling her what to think about the opposite sex. She knew from her own dating experiences and friendships with men that these experts didn't always get it right. So she decided to talk to actual guys about their actual sexual preferences. She enlisted the help of a real-live man, her husband, Nima Badiey, and sent out an online survey to about 300 men asking them what they wished their wives and girlfriends knew about seduction, foreplay, oral sex, masturbation, intercourse, sexual positions, body image, and more. Their candid answers formed the basis for the book *What Men Really Want in Bed: The Surprising Secrets Men Wish Women Knew About Sex.*

Yes, there were secrets. And yes, those secrets were surprising. Who would have expected, for example, that more than 50 percent of the men answering Cynthia's survey would admit to faking an orgasm? The relative anonymity of the Internet seemed to give guys the freedom to say things they might never say to their partners. Like: They want a partner who's enthusiastic about being in bed with them. They care about her pleasure. And they do want an emotional connection with the women they sleep with. (Most of the time.)

It seemed only fair to give guys a chance to hear from women.

And thus, the idea for *What Women Really Want in Bed* was born. This time, Cynthia convinced her longtime friend Dana Fredsti, a talented writer in her own right, to join her as coauthor. (Cynthia's husband wasn't relegated to the sidelines, of course, but more on that later.)

> **"To me, it's more important that they act like they want to be with ME and that I'm the most beautiful person in the world to them. That's orgasmic."**
>
> **Elizabeth, 36, business owner**

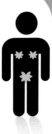

Using an online survey tool, we broadened the original survey to reach as many women as we could. We sent it to every woman we knew who wouldn't be offended—about 450—and then asked them to forward it to *their* friends. We sent it to the men who answered the survey for *What Men Really Want in Bed* and asked them to forward it to their girlfriends, wives, and female friends. We actually don't know how many women received the survey, but in the end, about 300 women responded.

Before we go any further, we need to trot out the caveat Cynthia used for the last book: This was by *no* means a scientific survey. Neither Cynthia nor Dana is a sociologist, psychologist, or scientist. (Dana is, however, a published mystery writer, which we thought made her uniquely qualified for the task of exploring the female psyche.) We're just writers with insatiable curiosity and dirty minds. Oh, we did try to bring in an anthro-pologist friend to vet our questions and help us design the survey—but when it turned out that he was hoping to turn our lighthearted list into a 500-question survey for a scientific treatise, we agreed to go our separate ways. We ended up asking women similar ques-tions to the ones Cynthia asked in *What Men Really Want in Bed*—and then we asked them some questions to which we thought guys would want to know the answers.

We got answers, all right. Pages and pages of candid, revealing answers, some hilarious, and some heartbreaking. In fact, there were so many excellent comments that we had no idea where to start. If not for Dana's boyfriend, David Fitzgerald, who organized hundreds of quotations into some sem-blance of order, we would still be sifting through them. We like to think that David enjoyed the task; after all, it wasn't like we were asking him to sort mathematical equations.

The women who answered our survey ranged in age from 22 to 70. They came from all walks of life and all professions. We had bankers, coffee baristas, stay-at-home moms, teachers, and executives. Given the nature of the topic, some of them wanted to keep some semblance of anonymity, so we let them choose pseudonyms—which will explain why some of the names you see are rather fanciful. We also let them name either their real profession or the job they'd like to have, so when you see someone quoted who's a "professional water-skier," know that it's quite possible she's not.

Some of the questions were multiple choice, and to those we received quantifiable data that SurveyMonkey.com analyzed for us (ah, the beauty of the Internet!), and those data are reflected in the pretty charts you see scattered throughout the book, courtesy of Cynthia's husband, Nima. (See! We told you he wouldn't be relegated to the sidelines. His stint as a management consultant was worth something.) That analysis showed us, for example, that exactly 73.4 percent of the women who responded to our survey wish that they were having *more* sex; 25.9 percent are perfectly satisfied, and 0.6 percent (one woman, that is) wish they were having less.

The takeaway from all this data and pages of comments? Women love sex. Women want sex. Women want *more* sex. But they want you to listen to them and show an interest in what they crave in the sack. That, we hope, is why you're reading this book. Use it to open up the lines of communication with your gal. Drop a couple of statistics into conversation, and ask her what she thinks. Read her a few of the more outrageous quotations. Use it to segue into a conversation about your own sex life. We firmly believe in the acronym OYMSYP (Open Your Mouth, Solve Your Problem). In other words, most issues could probably be solved if men and women just were honest with each other about what they want and need, instead of relying on assumptions, polls of their friends, or even the Internet. But until that happens, try listening to what real women have to say. So start reading, and start talking.

> **"Every woman is different—take the time to find out what we like, and don't slack off on the romance or trying to impress us in bed."**
>
> **Vanessa, 35, administrator**

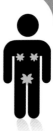

How to Find Out What *Your* Woman Wants in Bed

If there's one thing we hope you learn from this book, it's that, like snowflakes, no two women are alike. But that's where the metaphor ends. Because though some women will melt at your touch, others are unlike snowflakes and will remain frosty unless you take the time to find out what turns them on. Be willing to put the time into each step, from that first meeting to that delicious period when you're seducing each other and getting warmed up with some tantalizing foreplay, through to the joys of the main event, and the blissful period afterward. If you pace yourself and keep the lines of communication open, odds are you'll achieve a greater intimacy with your partner throughout your relationship—and have some truly mind-blowing sex as well!

If there's one point we took away after reading the survey responses (and hope *you'll* take away after reading this book), it's that despite many similarities, each woman has her own specific needs and wants when it comes to sex. It would be convenient if they all came with an owner's manual, but they don't. So the only way you can figure out what *your* woman wants in bed is to pay attention to her signals and cues . . . and talk to her. Use this book as a starting point. Ask her where she falls on the spectrum of responses. See what her reaction is to some of the comments. With any luck, your discussion will get her thinking about sex and turn into something more . . . "actionable," to use some horrible business jargon. Call it "mental foreplay," because that old saying is true: 99 percent of good sex happens between the ears.

Chapter 2

Fabulous Foreplay

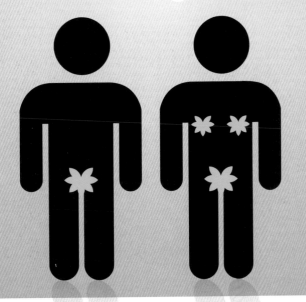

Is your idea of foreplay a quick round of tonsil hockey, followed by disrobing and the main event, in short order? Or are you one of those more sensitive types who really wants to know how to get his woman all hot and bothered before moving on to other activities?

If you're one of the former, we're here to tell you that while there's a place for the quickie—an activity that most women enjoy, *once in a while*—you'd do a lot better if you mastered the art of the sexual warm-up. If you don't believe us, read the rest of this chapter.

But if you need no convincing—you love sending your woman into a state of crazy desire before you do the deed—then this chapter will help you take your foreplay skills to new heights.

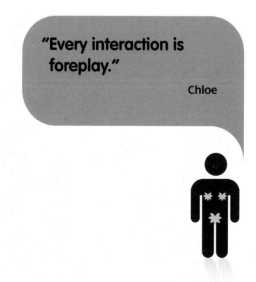

"Every interaction is foreplay."

Chloe

What Women Wish Men Knew about Foreplay

Foreplay is a crucial part of sex. But don't take our word for it. Read what the women in our survey had to say.

It's Not Optional

"Yeah, yeah, yeah," you're saying. "Foreplay's nice, but not totally necessary. I can be ready in 10 seconds, and she can, too!" Sorry, guys. Foreplay isn't a suggestion. It's a nonnegotiable part of sex. As Cynthia likes to say, "You gotta warm up the pan before you put the meat in!" Sure, you could slap your sausage in a cold skillet, but the cooking process is going to take a lot longer. (And with that, we'll stop this metaphor.) You get our drift: To most women, foreplay is important and necessary. "It's not a step you can skip and be successful," says Shelley, a 38-year-old artist. Some women even went so far as to say that it has emotional implications.

"Foreplay is mandatory for a woman to feel loved," says Elizabeth, a 36-year-old business owner. "It's part of the sexual package!"

In fact, several women emphasized that they don't see foreplay as separate from sex. As Nara, a 41-year-old massage therapist, puts it, "It's very important to the entire act of sexual congress." Adds Sophie, a 45-year-old designer, "It's not a preamble to be rushed."

Stacey, a 33-year-old marketing professional, was blunt. "Sex is not fun for a woman unless there's foreplay involved," she says. "Otherwise, we sort of feel like it's all about the man!"

But there's an even more important reason for making sure that foreplay's on the menu: Many women need it if they're going to climax. "I will never come without foreplay," says Ellen, 37, who manages a team of web developers.

Don't Rush It!

Okay. You get it. Foreplay is as vital to women as control of the television remote is to guys. But the other thing you have to know is that for best results, foreplay can't be hurried. Take your time, guys. Over and over, the women in our survey advised men to go slow. "Longer is better," says Judy, a 59-year-old clinical researcher. In other words, pawing her for two minutes before trying to jump her bones isn't going to cut it. "It doesn't have to last two hours, but rushing through it doesn't work," says 25-year-old Alina. Marla, a 44-year-old singer, puts it more succinctly: "The quick grope doesn't get us in the mood."

One of the reasons is anatomy. "Women take a lot longer to be ready than men do," says 32-year-old Alli, "so it's almost impossible to spend too long on foreplay." And she's right: women can take between 10 and 20 minutes to become aroused. That might be what Cari, a 26-year-old administrative assistant, means when she says, "We know you want to get there, but so do we, and foreplay is our time!"

Set the Mood

Hopefully, you already know that most women aren't like the drunken coeds on *Girls Gone Wild* and are *not* going to shimmy out of their tops and show you their hooters at the drop of a hat . . . or the pop of a beer bottle cap. But in case you have unrealistic, media-induced expectations, trust us when we tell you that most women want you to take the time to set the mood. Here are a few tips, but be sure to check out the secrets of seduction advice in the appendix!

> "It's important to set the right mood, being sweet and ge.ently with touching, caressing, and kissing."
> **Jeester, 36, human resources consultant**

> "If you take care of yourself and try to look nice and are well groomed, we will notice and think you are much more attractive and sexy . . . and be *much* more likely to have sex with you. We try to look as beautiful as possible for you . . . dress nice, makeup, shave, the whole nine yards. It's nice if the guy does the same. And being a gentleman and giving a compliment or two goes a long way in regards to getting in our pants! We want the romance, but we also want some raunchy sex!!!"
> **Heather, 25, executive assistant**

> "Good sex starts hours before you even get to the point of taking off clothes. Good preparation ensures a good time. A little tease and denial earlier in the timeline can jump-start the process."
> **Ginger, 38, project manager**

And remember that even if she feels wet, she may not be psychologically ready for you to enter her. As authors Cathy Winks and Anne Semans point out in *The Good Vibrations Guide to Sex*, "Few of us experience sexual arousal as though our bodies were space-ships moving inexorably from one discrete launching phase to another as we lift off toward a guaranteed orgasm. People need to *desire* sex to enjoy *having* sex." We'd suggest you keep a copy of this quotation in your nightstand. Or just keep repeating to yourself, "Her body is *not* a spaceship."

In other words, don't be surprised if it takes a while for her to get warmed up both physically *and* mentally. "If you think it's been going for too long, it's probably not long enough, so keep it going," advises Katia, a 34-year-old financial executive, expressing a sentiment that was common among our survey respondents. And there aren't any shortcuts—foreplay is one activity where less isn't more. "It needs to go on as long as it needs to go on," says Bryn, a 41-year-old secretary.

How will you know when you've gone on long enough? Watch and listen for her cues. Foreplay should "last until the woman's ready to move on—she'll let you know," says Julie, a 43-year-old artist and writer. "Let the woman start begging to go to the next step," says Troy, a 29-year-old lawyer. Cari was more specific: "Continue foreplay until I jump your bones. Let me set the pace."

But fear not: You won't be fooling around for hours on end (hopefully) without getting rewarded for your troubles. Indulging in drawn-out foreplay "just makes the women want you more," says Katia. So spend some time on it. Stretch it out. Adds Rose, a 30-year-old teacher: "I wish men knew that pacing leads to pleasure." Even a woman you've been with for several years might need some priming. "The longer you do it, the more it gets us going," says Blair, a 27-year-old lawyer. "And don't just do it in the beginning of a relationship. Even two years in, make foreplay hot and sexy and not just about getting it on." (Your authors would say that this is true throughout a relationship, not just two years in!)

So if you're not rushing it, what *should* you be doing? Several women gave specific advice on how to draw things out for maximum foreplay fun:

"Slow, teasing actions are the BEST!"
Richelle, 47, attorney

"Use a soft and lingering touch. Don't rush it or appear impatient."
Maureen, 45, archeologist

"It's fun! It can be great if it's long and lingering. Don't be bored and rush through."
Helena, 39, professor

"Take your time, but don't stay too long in one place."
Esra, age and occupation withheld

"Enjoy the journey. The best foreplay I had was being kissed head to toe."
Karen, 35, student

"It doesn't have to slowly rise before sex. Arousal that climbs and slows, then climbs again is the best for me."
Teresa, 33, marketer

"Take it easy! Going harder or faster isn't going to make me orgasm faster! Slow down and be a bit gentler."
Lulu, 35, defense attorney

"Do it for a real amount of time, with interest—no, with fascination!"
Helen, 48, executive

You get the idea. Besides, the fact of the matter is that once you get to the point where you're engaging in foreplay, the outcome is usually clear. As Leslie, a 32-year-old national account specialist, puts it, "Don't rush. I'm not going anywhere."

But Sometimes, a Quickie Is Okay

Now that we've drilled it into your heads that you shouldn't rush foreplay, we're going to qualify it: Foreplay doesn't need to take hours. Many women extol the virtues of getting right down to business. We all have fond memories of a simple morning goodbye kiss that turned into a passionate standing-up-against-the-wall encounter. Says Heather, a 25-year-old executive assistant, "Sometimes we want a lot of foreplay—sometimes it can be better than sex itself. Other times, we want to just skip foreplay and get naked for a quickie!" Michelle, a 36-year-old management consultant, agreed, and notes that you should trust your gal when she tells you to dispense with the preamble: "Although I LOVE foreplay, sometimes a quickie is okay, too! When I tell you that, I really mean it!"

And even if she does need some warming up, your woman may not need a lot of it. "I like foreplay, but sometimes guys think it has to last for hours," says Matilda, a 32-year-old pharmacist. "There are situations where you just want to do IT right away without waiting." Shannon, a 40-year-old travel writer, says, "If I'm ready to go, I'm ready to go," while Brooke reminds guys, "We don't necessarily need to come three times before sex!"

And yes, while foreplay is a necessary part of sex, to many women it's "just the appetizer," as, Paula, 55, puts it. "Sometimes the best foreplay is ripping my clothes off!" says Destiny (age and occupation not provided).

Don't Go Straight for Her Genitals

If you really want to get her warmed up, don't head straight for her breasts and her groin. A smart lover knows how to tease and tantalize. Touch as much of her body as possible before "going in for the goods" (Paris, 24, scientist) and "stay above the waist for some time" (Sarah, 47, attorney). Her entire body can be an erogenous zone—and that includes what's between her ears. Be creative and explore it. Make her genitals the *last* thing you go for, so that she's dying for your intimate touch.

"Most women aren't race cars—they can't go from zero to 60 in 10 seconds," explains Roxanne, a 45-year-old writer. "Please spend some time getting us warmed up. It doesn't have to be hours. Just don't always head straight between my legs before paying attention to the other parts of my body (including my brain)."

Other specific tips from our survey respondents:

> "Start with light, gentle touching all over my body. Surprise me with where your hands go. Don't just thrust your fingers down my pants during the first minute."
> **Abbey, 30, designer**

> "Touch me everywhere, not just one place, assuming, 'Well, I checked off kissing the breasts, so now it's sex time!'"
> **Carrie, 28, entrepreneur**

"Don't head straight for the nipples or the clitoris. Teasing for a while lets me build up steam, whereas going straight for the hot buttons can be irritating!"
Inara, 46, writer

As we've said before, drawing out foreplay works to your benefit. "Men need to tease more," says Summer, a 27-year-old TV advertising executive. "If they were to touch everywhere and avoid the obvious erogenous zones as long as possible, the anticipation alone would make for a much more intense arousal."

Scarlet, a 34-year-old chef, put it this way: "The slower and more lingering you are (as opposed to rushing straight to the crotch), the hotter we'll get and the more likely it will be that you'll be initiating further activity."

Love Her Tender

So how should you approach a woman's body? Be gentle. It's fine to be passionate; it's not so fine to be rough and insensitive. Don't treat her breasts as "pinball machine controls" (as Jackie remembered one man doing) or her nipples as "radio channel dials" (a particularly painful memory for Inara). And when you're going farther south, remember the words of Lula, a 30-year-old librarian: "The clitoris is extremely sensitive, and if the guy attacks it right off the bat, it freaking hurts! Start slow and gentle."

Most women do crave the feel of your hands during foreplay—and why not, seeing as how the skin is the largest organ of the human body. That's why Elizabeth, a 28-year-old

advertising sales manager, advises, "Don't stop touching me. Skin is incredibly sensitive for women."

Gentle touching "goes a long way," as Violet, a 40-year-old scientist, says, but make sure that you always keep the recipient in mind. Women have a sixth sense when it comes to selfishness. "Touch me to make me feel something," Ava says, "not because you want to touch that part of me."

Most important, a gentle touch will put your partner at ease, instead of making her feel like she needs to be constantly defending herself against full-frontal assault. "It's just as important that a woman feel relaxed as it is that she feel turned on," says Keite, a 32-year-old office manager.

Be Creative

Variety is the spice of life, as the old saying goes—and it's also the spice of foreplay. Getting your woman worked up isn't "paint-by-numbers," as Erika, a 50-year-old writer and teacher, puts it, so vary your routine and try new moves. Don't always go with what you know will get her off, although, of course, "you can end there," says Dawn, a 29-year-old public relations executive. Don't be afraid to try new things. "It's more fun if you don't always do the same things in the same order," Mae, a 31-year-old graduate student, comments. Adds Vanessa, a 35-year-old administrator: "I get frustrated when it starts to feel predictable."

The chances are good that what excites your woman will vary, depending on a host of factors. "What turns me on is always different," says Sara, a 30-year-old engineer. "Sometimes suggestive talk is the best. Sometimes it's a back massage, sometimes it's when he massages my feet and works his way up. Sometimes just looking into each other's eyes is the best foreplay. And sometimes I just like it rough and dirty."

So how do you go about mixing up your moves? We know you're fond of your little man, but try having sex for an hour with a woman *without* involving your penis. What would you do then? What would you focus on? Be creative. This is where adult toys can come in handy. "'Foreplay' assumes intercourse is the goal," says Annette, a 44-year-old manager. "But it's not always. Women pleasure women very nicely without a penis."

No matter what, stay tuned in to her cues. "When we signal that what you're doing isn't working, that is not a sign to go back to the same spot with more vim and vigor," advises Carissa, a 34-year-old communications consultant. "Give it up and try something else!"

Listen and Learn

This brings us to our next tip: During foreplay, pay close attention to your partner's signals, both verbal and nonverbal. "We give you cues as to what's working and what's not," says Ulla, a 25-year-old performer. Yet it seems that, at times, men are oblivious to those cues. "Sometimes men have absolutely no sensitivity to feedback—almost as if you're not even there," says Hailey.

And if you're a little rusty with your ESP? "Listen to what a woman likes (by what she says or the sounds she makes), and if she doesn't communicate it clearly, ask her what she likes," advises 34-year-old Jennifer, who works for a nonprofit organization.

You Should Be Enjoying It, Too!

All the tips and techniques in the world won't help you with foreplay if you're not having fun (and, judging from what Cynthia discovered in writing *What Men Really Want in Bed*, most men are), if you're just going through the motions, or if you view it as a chore. Over and over, the women in our survey said they wanted guys to enjoy themselves and relish the art of arousal. "The more you love us and our bodies, the more we'll get into it," says Ilea, a 24-year-old actuarial analyst. In fact, the word *fun* was one women used repeatedly. "It shouldn't be so terribly serious," said Jyllian, a 44-year-old engineer and mother. "Laughter works quite well."

Jenny, a 30-year-old medical office manager, sums it up perhaps the best when she says, "The word has *play* in it for a reason. Bringing in some fun and playfulness puts me at ease, and then I might be more likely to experiment later."

What Kind of Foreplay Gets Women the Hottest?

So let's get down to basics: Keeping in mind that every woman is different, what specifically is the best thing to do if you want to get her going?

Focus on Her Brain

Although we know it does a lot for *you*, just getting a woman naked won't necessarily turn her on. Her horniness often depends on psychological factors: how comfortable she is with you, whether she's had a good or bad day at work, or how tired she is. Nearly 28 percent of women said that the type of foreplay that gets them the hottest completely depends on their mood and the situation. Second, around 23 percent specifically called out "mental" foreplay as the surest spark for lighting their fire. Foreplay "doesn't always have to be physical," says Alicia, who didn't give her age or occupation. "Working my imagination is sometimes a bigger turn-on."

For many women, mental foreplay means flirting and other types of suggestive talk. "If you talk dirty, we might actually like it," says Heather, a 37-year-old marine biologist; others find intimacy and intellectual connection enticing. Several women gave suggestions on what mental foreplay could entail:

> "Mental sparring? Mental debate? Best foreplay."
> **Daisy, 40, stay-at-home mom**

> "Talking, when there is a true communication, that sense of 'Yes, exactly!' but with the undercurrent of attraction and flirtation."
> **Rachel, 45, entrepreneur**

> "If you want me, I should be able to feel it."
> **Francesca, 39, education professional**

> "I need to feel special and desired."
> **Michelle, 44, stay-at-home mom**

> "Engage my brain first. Make me feel like you really want me and can't control your feelings around me."
> **Allison, age and occupation withheld**

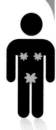

"The brain is the sexiest organ on a woman."
Murphy, 60, artist

What type of foreplay gets you the hottest? What's your biggest turn-on?

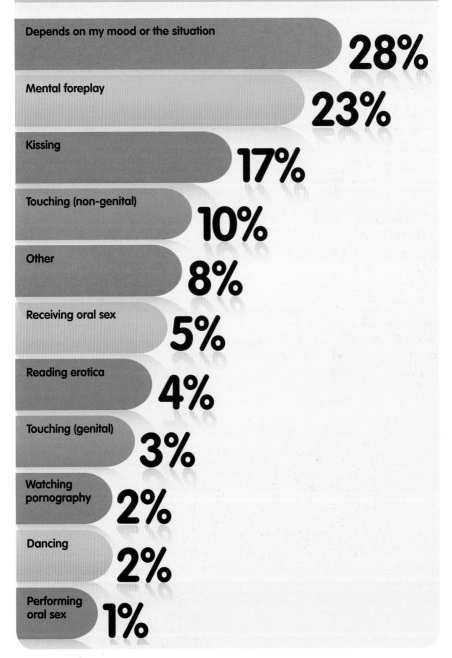

Depends on my mood or the situation **28%**

Mental foreplay **23%**

Kissing **17%**

Touching (non-genital) **10%**

Other **8%**

Receiving oral sex **5%**

Reading erotica **4%**

Touching (genital) **3%**

Watching pornography **2%**

Dancing **2%**

Performing oral sex **1%**

Note: Percentages may not equal 100% due to rounding.

"It's not all about the genitals for me. I like foreplay in my brain more."
Emily, 30, attorney

"It doesn't always have to be physical. Working my imagination is sometimes a greater turn-on."
Alicia, age and occupation withheld

"The brain is the sexiest organ on a woman." **Murphy, 60, artist**

"Mind over body."
Beth, 43, designer

"Every interaction is foreplay."
Chloe, age and occupation withheld

A major tactical error in this department? Waiting until you're between the sheets to engage her brain. "I think men underestimate the importance of mental foreplay," says Sunny, a 36-year-old project manager. "Or maybe they don't realize that this type of foreplay can start *way* in advance of the actual act with things like racy emails while you're work."

Michelle, a 35-year-old marketing project manager, agreed. "It can start hours in advance with a look, a light touch, a whispered suggestion in the ear," she says.

Which brings us to one final word: Make sure that whispered suggestion is a romantic one. Sylvia, a 48-year-old marketing representative, reminds guys that hot mental foreplay isn't "telling me how 'we need to get naked because it's been two weeks.' Thank you, Mr. Calendar."

Master the Art of Kissing

Kissing says a lot about who you are and what you'll be like as a lover. (Hence the phrase "as above, so below.") Women know that a bad kisser will probably be bad in bed. On the other hand, a good kisser almost guarantees his chances of moving to the next level. Perhaps that's why nearly 17 percent of our survey takers named kissing as their favorite type of foreplay. And this holds true even if you're in a long-term relationship. The most eloquent comment on the subject came from Caroline, a 29-year-old teacher, who says: "Making out is an art, and after you've had sex for the first time, it often becomes a lost art. Don't lose it. It keeps you young, heightens anticipation, and gives us time to get our motors purring."

So what type of kiss do women like? Just as you shouldn't dive straight for her genitals, don't start a make-out session with your mouth wide opening and your tongue protruding. (Shudder.) Start slow and gentle, and then build in intensity. Explore her mouth with your tongue; use it to show her how you'd like to make love to her. Express yourself through your kiss. In fact, 61 percent of our survey respondents prefer kisses that are deep and lingering. "Kissing can go on for a long time," says Judy, 36, a teacher. Gentle kisses came in second, followed by kisses that are "short and sweet" (although at least one of your coauthors, who dated—briefly—a guy who refused to part his lips while kissing, would put this dead last) and "vigorous." The least favorite type of kiss?

Seventy-three percent said that a wet and sloppy kiss is their least favorite, so keep your spit in your mouth, guys—not her face. To recap, go for the deep and lingering, avoid the wet and sloppy.

Use the Power of Touch

When it comes to hot foreplay, we're here to extol the virtues of touch. And by "touch," we don't mean groping her privates—only 2.6 percent cited genital touching as their biggest turn-on. Think instead about caressing her all over her body, from the top of her head to her toes. Stroke your fingers up and down her arms. Kiss her in the hollow of her neck. Hug her tightly and let her feel the heat from your body.

Cari says that her favorite type of foreplay is "random touching, like hugging, kissing the back of my neck, wrapping his arms around me, and holding my hand." Some forms of touch are more unique: Arianna, a 33-year-old who describes herself as a "household engineer," says she loves having the bottom of her feet touched lightly, just to the point of tickling. This isn't surprising, considering the concentration of nerve endings in the toes and the soles of the feet.

You won't be surprised, of course, to learn that many women find a massage an excellent precursor to sex. (Probably because it offers a legitimate excuse for taking off clothes, a fact that one of your coauthors used to her benefit in her shady past. Now, however, said coauthor would rather pay someone for a massage so that she can fall asleep without feeling guilty.) However, that's not always the case. Some women can't stand to get massages. Bryn notes, "My husband is a licensed massage therapist, so massaging is a turnoff because it makes me think of his clients. I love men's hands, though, and I love to have my neck, throat, hair, shoulders, and breasts touched."

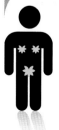

> "I love men's hands, though, and I love to have my neck, throat, hair, shoulders, and breasts touched."
>
> **Bryn, 41, secretary**

Don't think that sexual touching is always out of the question, however. Several women mentioned touching that leads to oral sex (receiving, not giving it). But the prevailing sentiment was that men need a little more skill at manual labor. "Learn how to masturbate me," advises January, a 45-year-old paralegal, while Nana, a 37-year-old marketing manager, wants her man to "spend more time stimulating my clitoris during foreplay while kissing." If you're going to go this route, don't grope blindly about. "They should read sex books about pleasing women—seriously," says Paige. "There are some technical things they should know, like where the G-spot and clitoris are."

And don't discount the power of touch to express your desire. Heather, a 25-year-old executive assistant, finds that her motors really start revving "when you start kissing heavily, and just can't keep your hands off each other and want to rip each other's clothes off!"

Oral Sex Equals Sex

Only about 5 percent of our survey respondents named oral sex as the act that makes them randiest. That's because for many women, cunnilingus (and to a lesser extent, fellatio) is the main event, not a warm-up. As Annette comments, "It depends on the situation, but I think it is important to understand that 'foreplay' assumes intercourse is the ultimate act. It should not be. For me, oral sex, either receiving or performing, *is* sex."

If you're going to use oral sex to warm her up, learn how to do it right (and our respondents will give you tips in the next chapter). Annie, a 62-year-old writer, thinks that men should learn "how to give cunnilingus so it really feels good and brings the woman to orgasm before intercourse. My first husband always pressed too hard; my second husband obviously didn't like it. Between them, there were a few real experts, but they were few and far between. Sigh."

Or as Roxy, a 31-year-old administrator, puts it more bluntly: "It's not a piece of bubblegum. You don't *chew* it."

Choreplay

Men, don't underestimate the erotic potential of household chores. Help her out at home, and ecstasy will be your reward. And if you think you're already doing your bit, well, trust us, you're probably not, according to numerous surveys. Stacey, a 33-year-old marketing professional who's also the mother of a preschooler, says it all: "To me, these days, foreplay is anything he does that takes some of the burden off me. If I come home and he did a load of laundry and started dinner and offers to do bath- and bedtime that night, he's getting some, because I won't be exhausted at the end of the day. Unfortunately for men, they don't usually understand that!"

Her Body Is a Wonderland: Her Erogenous Zones

When you hear the word *erogenous*, we bet you're thinking "genitals." Instead, we'd suggest you keep in mind that the actual definition of *erogenous*—"especially sensitive to sexual stimulation"—doesn't say anything about penises or vaginas, which opens up a whole new world of possibilities! Need examples? Take a look at some favorite (nongenital) erogenous zones.

Her Face

At the top of the list was the face—and not just her lips. "I love little kisses on my forehead since I'm (ideally) shorter than the guy," says Carrie, the 28-year-old entrepreneur. "I love when he bends down and give me a short and sweet kiss on my forehead. Just makes me feel like a special little princess."

Her Neck

Next up: the neck, which Sunny, 36, calls "far and away" her favorite erogenous zone. Annette, 42, gushes that "a slightly aggressive neck kiss or nibble during sex is incredible."

Her Breasts

Breasts ranked third on our list. "During passionate kissing, I have two 'go' buttons: my left and my right breasts," says Casi. We were a little surprised to see that they ranked right above the lips and mouth, given that so many women mentioned kissing as their favorite type of foreplay. But it makes sense: A woman's breasts—particularly her nipples—are packed with nerve endings. "My breasts in general aren't sensitive, but the nipples are, especially with pressure from biting or pinching," says Jennifer, the 34-year-old nonprofit worker.

When you become aroused from nipple stimulation, your body releases a hormone called oxytocin. This wonderful chemical is sometimes called the "cuddle hormone" because your body also releases it during breastfeeding, which promotes bonding with your baby.

Her Other Erogenous Zones

Move down her body—you'll be surprised at the hot spots you'll find. Women in our survey mentioned collarbones ("Oh, yeah!" Karen, 35), lower back ("Surprisingly sensitive," Beth, 43, designer), the upper arm right before the armpit, the inside of the elbow, the delicate skin inside the forearm, hands, and of course, feet ("A good foot rub constitutes foreplay," Marisol, 66, writer). Several women mentioned the backs of their knees, and indeed, because the skin here is thin, the nerves are closer to the surface and more easily stimulated.

Wondering where your woman's hot buttons are? If you're not sure, ask her. But you can't go wrong paying attention to her entire body. Whether they love a "firm but sweet" touch (Elizabeth, 54, actress) or a light caress ("Use it, boys!" Grape, 32, model/actress), women just want you to touch them. "I love being touched about 99 percent of the time and over 99 percent of my body," says 46-year-old writer Inara. And be creative: "Originality can trump my preferences," advises Ginger, a 38-year-old project manager.

But for the last—and most eloquent—word on touching and erogenous zones, we have to go to Helena, the 39-year-old professor. "I think amazing touching just about anywhere is the absolute best and a total turn-on," she says. "I love just being naked with someone I trust and am attracted to and touching each other everywhere."

Foreplay: What Not to Do

So we've convinced you to devote time and energy to foreplay. But there *are* certain mistakes you should definitely avoid if you're trying to get her in the mood.

First off, take a close look at the chart below. Each of these missteps risks sending your woman for the door. In fact, for many women, all of these are deal-breakers. "I can only specify one?" asks Bryn, the 41-year-old secretary. "Any of these things kills my mood: being rushed, if he's bored or passive, or if he's doing the same thing every time."

Here are some of the specific tips we got on foreplay gaffes.

Remember That Cleanliness Is Next to Sexiness

Sure, a woman might admire Matthew McConaughey's abs. But unless you *are* Matthew McConaughey, you probably won't be able to get away with his alleged refusal to wear deodorant. We'll put it bluntly. Nothing—and we mean nothing—will turn a woman off faster than a guy who stinks. In our survey, 31 percent (a majority) of our respondents chose poor hygiene as their biggest turnoff.

If you start fooling around, what would turn you off?

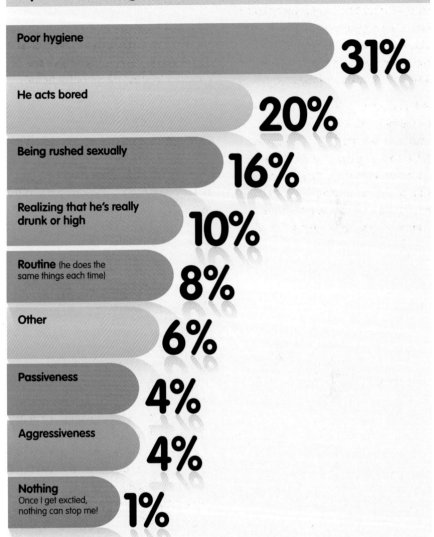

Poor hygiene — 31%

He acts bored — 20%

Being rushed sexually — 16%

Realizing that he's really drunk or high — 10%

Routine (he does the same things each time) — 8%

Other — 6%

Passiveness — 4%

Aggressiveness — 4%

Nothing Once I get exctied, nothing can stop me! — 1%

Note: Percentages may not equal 100% due to rounding.

So if you know (or hope) you're going to be fooling around, wash up first. "For God's sake, let's all have a shower beforehand!" exclaims Dawn, the 42-year-old domestic executive. Adds 45-year-old entrepreneur Rachel, "If I get a whiff of something that smells bad, ewwww!"

Don't Forget That There's Another Person Involved

Acting bored. Rushing her. Implying that her needs aren't important. All of these gaffes will put you in the penalty box. Alex, a 35-year-old college professor, gets turned off and frustrated "when he's not responsive— he keeps touching me wrong or too hard, or has a problem with me weighing in."

Heather, a 31-year-old song artist, says that her biggest foreplay turnoff is "when it's all about him and he treats me like a blow-up doll."

Don't Go on Autopilot

Say you've got a signature move that seems to really light her jets. Or you've been with her a while and know her body and its responses like the back of your own hand. Well, guess what? After a while, those tried-and-true tricks will stop getting you results. "I get really turned off by routine sex," says Ava. "Him heaving his body on top of me is supposed to turn me on?"

Just like in the beginning of a relationship, when everything's new and fresh and exciting, don't forget the element of surprise. Otherwise, "I know what to expect and I just get really bored," as Carissa says.

Think of it this way: Experts say that taking a different route to work every once in a while forges new connections in your brain and keeps you young. The same thing applies to pleasure, so mix it up.

Keep Your Past to Yourself

Seraphin, a 40-year-old technology strategist, says that once she starts fooling around, the thing that will turn her off is "if he mentions anything about other women he slept with, e.g., what they liked."

Which brings us to our next point. We shouldn't really have to remind you about this, but we will anyway. Remember that signature move we mentioned previously? Remember how it sent your college girlfriend over the edge? Great. Remember it, but *don't talk about it while you're fooling around with your current partner*. "This always worked for Bambi" is not a phrase that is going to help your cause.

We're not saying that your past has to be a black hole of mystery and enigma. In fact, one of the joys and great reliefs of strong long-term relationships is that you're comfortable and confident enough to talk to your partner about past relationships without either party being threatened. (Cynthia and her husband find these discussions to be sources of great hilarity.) Even so, it's probably best to avoid going there while you're in the act.

Good Things Come to Those Who Wait

We don't want to leave you with the impression that foreplay is a minefield. Quite the opposite: women love foreplay as much as you do—and we know that you do, as Cynthia discovered in her research for *What Men Really Want in Bed*. In case you need more convincing, here are some closing thoughts:

"The more you put me off, the hotter I'll get."
Amy, 30, scientist

"The longer you spend on it and the more effort you put into it, the more you'll increase the pleasure for both partners during intercourse."
Pearl, 22, chemist

"Men need to understand how powerful foreplay is. If he does it, he can probably have whatever he wants."
Vicky, 43, professional water-skier

"If you'd just give us 10 to 15 minutes of foreplay, we'll give you anything you want after that. (At least I would!)"
Adrienne, 33, graduate student

"Know how much it enhances the sexual experience for both the woman and the man."
Liz, 36, physician

"The more excited he is about my body and pleasing me, the more excited I'll get, the better I'll feel, and the more I'll want to return the favor."
Camilla, 25, advertising manager

"Don't rush, put in a little effort, and you'll get a lot of enthusiasm in return!"
Dawn, 42, domestic executive

"Try it. It works."
Morgan, 26, graduate student

But we thought the best (the most colorful and topical, at least) argument for foreplay came from Roxie, a 35-year-old communications professional: "Think of it as a ROI: return on investment. It's best to thoroughly check out *all* of the stocks and bonds available (every inch of her body), and see which areas respond to your investment/ attention. Understand that some fluctuate and change, ebb and flow, and that's part of the 'thrill.' Stay focused, keep studying, and expect nothing less than for the market to completely explode in your favor. You'll enjoy the riches, I promise."

Chapter 3

Hands On

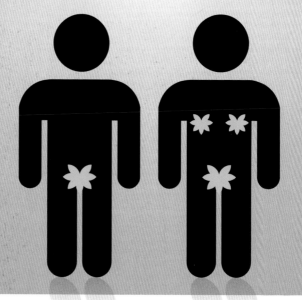

Women appreciate being in good hands. Think of the possibilities of your magic touch: running your hands through her hair, fingering her lips, softly scratching down her back, caressing every inch of her skin, lifting her in your arms, grabbing her butt, and pulling her into you. Women crave your hands on their body in every way imaginable, from the most delicate butterfly kiss of your fingertips to your strongest love embrace. But don't take our word for it. Hear it in their own words.

> "Always be touching me somewhere."
>
> Nara, 41, massage therapist

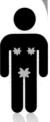

What Women Wish Men Knew about Using Their Hands

To paraphrase Billy Idol: "More! More! More!" That's right. Women can't get enough of your touch, guys, whether you're giving them light caresses or firm grips in the right places. Before, during, and after sex, the right kind of touch can be the difference between a night of passion or a pass on the night.

"They should use their hands more!" exclaims Brianna, a 30-year-old marketing specialist—along with 99 percent of the woman we surveyed. Thirty-year-old Sarah, a salesperson, notes that "most women need additional stimulation to have an orgasm, so it's a good thing."

In fact, women can't seem to emphasize enough how much they crave touch all over their bodies. "Women really like it!" Katherine, a 38-year-old manager, assures us. "It's sexy to be touched," says researcher Z.B., 27. Christina, a 32-year-old working in marketing and advertising, agrees: "It's a turn-on and shouldn't be forgotten during intercourse."

A good lover learns to take the time to explore her whole body, not just the most obvious choices. Here are a few tips.

Don't Go Straight for the Genitals—Touch Her All Over

It's amazing how many women complain that their partners never pay attention to any parts of their body other than their nipples and vagina. Your woman doesn't have an "on" switch, guys. She needs to be tantalized and teased . . . and that starts in areas other than the hot spots. "Touch doesn't need to center on the erogenous zones," says Karen, a 35-year-old student. "Grab the back of my neck when you kiss me, stroke my hair, caress my body, hold my hands and wrists."

Advertising sales manager Elizabeth, 28, agrees: "Don't go for my genitals and breasts right away! Touch the rest of my body to get me stimulated; butt, neck, back, hips, legs." As Ava says, "Just keep touching me somewhere."

The good news is that your patience in paying attention to her entire body will pay off. Blair, a 27-year-old lawyer, says, "It feels really good to have hands touching me all over and feeling the strength of a man's hands, yet the gentle side, too." And Kelly, 32, a wildlife biologist and dance fitness instructor, has the best news of all: "Make me purr. Once I'm turned on, every part of me is an erogenous zone!"

Start Slow and Build Up

If you knew only this one lovemaking secret and nothing else, you would still be a better lover than one who knows everything else *but doesn't know this*: It's all about the buildup. Here's the formula:

> "Go slowly and start out super lightly—less is WAY more when you're first starting out. Building suspense = building desire."
> **Andrea, 40, administrative manager**

> "Start lightly and then add more pressure. Have the entire process go slowly."
> **Elizabeth, 32, mental health provider**

> "Light touches in the beginning . . . barely touching the skin. And as things heat up, so can the pressure and movement."
> **Chloe**

> "Give me more teasing. Make me want it."
> **Beth, 43, designer**

> "I like things to build up, so I don't want to be rushed into too much stimulation too soon. Indirect contact in the very beginning, light and slow in the middle, harder and faster once I'm excited."
> **Bryn, 41, secretary**

Keep in mind that flitting around her body like a hummingbird is not what we're talking about either. If you find something that works (and believe us, pay attention and she will let you know), stick to it. There's nothing more frustrating than feeling the slow surge of an impending orgasm, only to have it derailed when one's partner suddenly decides to totally change the area and rhythm. Twenty-nine-year-old Dawn, a public relations executive, counsels, "Take your time. Keep the rhythm. Don't change motions every five seconds. That's distracting." Daisy, a 40-year-old stay-at-home mom, adds, "It isn't about more stimulation, it's about the right stimulation at the right time."

Some women need time before actual penetration; it takes them a while to build to a point where they're ready for intercourse. Thirty-two-year-old Elli cautions, "Please don't put anything inside my vagina until I'm really turned on. Wait until I beg."

Be Gentle!

Yes, women crave the feeling of your hands on their body. What they *don't* crave is you pawing at them like an overeager puppy. Again, go easy, at least at first. As you would when giving a massage, start gently but firmly, and notice her cues. It's a dance where her responses will build on each other. "Light touches are almost always better," advises 30-year-old librarian Lulu. "If I want more, I'll say so." For 26-year-old actress Zelda, "light caresses and fingertips are always good"; similarly, 66-year-old writer Marisol says that "light stroking works best, except for backrubs."

Forty-five-old designer Sophie reminds lovers that the gentleness they crave isn't just physical. "I'm not an instrument," says Sophie. "Touching needs eye contact, warm smiles, and sounds. Emotional and mental interaction is essential." In other words, a guy can have the best technique in the world, but it can still fall flat if there's no effort at emotional and mental connection.

Although sometimes women do love to be manhandled, most of our respondents prefer subtlety. A light, teasing caress is often more stimulating than a rough squeeze. "Don't be too rough, unless I ask for it," says Liz, a 36-year-old physician.

In fact, coming on too strong may backfire on you. "We aren't dolls," says Judy, a 59-year-old clinical researcher, "and although we won't break, don't try to pretend we are jars with tight lids." This is especially true when it comes to her love button. Carrie, a 40-year-old scientist, says, "Sometimes my clitoris gets overstimulated and becomes *sore*. Don't be too rough early on or you may wear it out." There aren't any replacements for those parts, guys, so be gentle unless otherwise requested.

In addition to the clitoris, breasts are also frequently abused targets. We've met men who use what we call the "dough kneading" technique. Here's the thing: Breasts won't double in size no matter how hard or long you rub and squeeze them, and many women have very sensitive nipples, especially during ovulation or their periods. Paula, 55, lays down the law: "My breasts are not to be milked like a cow."

Twenty-nine-year-old teacher Caroline gives it to you straight: "Less is more, and we can always ask you for more. If you start out with too much pressure or motion, we have to tell you to slow down, and we'll hesitate about doing that because we're afraid to criticize your technique and hurt your feelings."

In addition to being gentle, take your time. Lulu, a 35-year-old defense attorney, wants you to "slow down and be a bit gentler." Twenty-six-year-old Cari, an administrative assistant, sums it up: "Slow and steady wins the race!"

Be Confident and Assertive

At the same time, don't be *too* gentle. (Oh, guys, you knew it wasn't *that* simple, right?) Gentle, yes—but firm. If you can master this balance, she'll be sighing about you to her friends tomorrow. Whether it is a massage or lovemaking (or, if you want to be *really* popular, both combined), no one wants flimsy, tepid strokes any more than they want to be jackhammered. So what's the secret? Jill, a 37-year-old executive, counsels, "Be firm, but not too aggressive." Susie, a 52-year-old marketing consultant, recommends "soft, gentle, firm probing in all directions." Marketing project manager Michelle, 35, may sum it up best when she says, "I want to feel handled, so be confident, firm, and assertive."

Mix It Up

Once you have the right touch and pacing, the other thing women want you to keep in mind is variety. Don't become predictable. Shannon, a 40-year-old travel writer, says, "Exploration is good. Don't always do the same thing." According to Alina, a 25-year-old academic, "It's best to change things up once in a while. Overstimulation of one area can have the opposite effect." So offer variety. Stay in one place for a while and move to another—the unexpected is what's fun. (Unless she's about to have an orgasm. In that case, keep doing what you're doing until you take her over the edge. We're talking about foreplay here.) "I shouldn't always get what I want when I want it," says Ginger, a 38-year-old project manager. "Denying something is equally as stimulating."

Remember That She Wants It as Much as You Do

Sometimes men forget that women enjoy and crave sex as much as they do. We're still living in a world where it's more acceptable for men to make the advances. It takes a lot of courage for many women to make their desires known.

> "I want it more than you think. I get sad and rejected when you shoot me down or ignore my subtle advances. I would like to try new things and new places, but I need a little help to start talking about these things."
> **Jenny, 28, medical office manager**

> "Fuck me good and hard and love me 'til the end . . . tease me, taste me, explore me, open me. I'll be your whore; I'll be your sweet. Tell me what you need and I'll give you me!"
> **Marla, 30, artist**

Some women want a mix of tender and passionate. Roxie, a 35-year-old communications professional, says, "Don't underestimate the light touch. Make it even more powerful by mixing it up with the firm and aggressive." And 29-year-old Ulla, a performer, points out that once you know the rules, you'll know when to break them. "Mix it up!" she says. "I usually like it gentle, but am often pleasantly surprised when he roughs it up!"

Listen to Her Cues

Confused about where and how much and when and what kind of pressure to use? Many women like Raena, a 52-year-old business owner, want you to "be aware of my feelings and what I want." Easier said than done? Forty-year-old Seraphin, 40, a technology strategist, sympathizes with your plight: "No wonder they say we want them to be mind readers," Seraphin sighs. "We really do." But all is not lost. Sara, a 30-year-old engineer, says it's really about creativity: "He needs to explore what I like, and be open-minded and inventive."

To do this, you need to pay attention to your partner's cues. And believe us, the average woman will be doing her best to let you know what does or does not work for her. "Let my hands guide you," says 33-year-old writer Gayle. This can mean a women will literally guide your hands to where she wants them to go, or, if she's too shy to do that, can also mean she'll touch you the way she'd like to be touched.

Meagen, a 37-year-old psychotherapist, advises you to "be gentle and pay attention to nonverbal cues," and she isn't alone. "Listen and observe my reactions, and if something looks to be working, stick with it," says Sheba, 35, a lawyer. "If it doesn't provoke a reaction, move on to something different." Pay attention to her expressions, too. "Start with light pressure and look at my face and anticipate if I want more," suggests 31-year-old administrator Roxy.

Don't get complacent, either. Just as all women are different, what pleasures an individual woman during one lovemaking session may leave her cold in the next. Annette, a 44-year-old manager, notes that "what worked yesterday may not work today. Pay attention to nonverbal cues, moaning, arching of the back, pulling away. Or simply ask me, 'Where?'"

Also important: If a woman tells you "no," pay attention. That's not a cue; it's an order. Marla, a 44-year-old singer, cautions, "No means no for certain practices and areas. It doesn't mean 'Wait until I'm really into it and you can do whatever you want.' Nothing kills the mood more than not respecting boundaries."

The lesson here is that your lover won't have a problem with you checking in with her; in fact, she may well be counting on it. Women like Casi want to remind you that the two of you are a team. "Ask what I would like, ask what feels good," she says. "Hey, we're doing this together, this intimate communication. I'll ask you how you like it. Don't be afraid to ask me."

Enjoy Yourself!

For most women, it's not just about their enjoyment and involvement; it's about yours, too. An actively engaged partner who's obviously having fun is much more of a turn-on than a guy who's only paying cursory attention to what he's doing. Be present and let her know you're as into her as she is to you. Roxanne, a 45-year-old writer, tells us, "If I sense that you like what you're doing and into turning me on, I'll be able to relax and enjoy it much more." As stay-at-home mom Michelle, 44, says, "Do it with passion. Touch. Feel. Enjoy. Have fun."

Push My Buttons (The Right Ways)

When it comes to the clitoris, there's no single way to touch her that trumps the rest. Yet, some techniques are more popular than others: The women in our survey generally like light pressure with a steady rhythm, or an indirect touch on either side of the clitoris. Some women don't have one favorite move: "It varies throughout the course of arousal," Elizabeth, a 32-year-old mental health provider tells us. "Everything I checked feels good at some point in the process."

The Most Popular Ways to Use Your Hands

Many of our survey respondents shared a specific clitoral technique that drives them wild. Here's a sampling of what rings their bells:

> "I like light little flicks or very gentle strokes on the clitoris, but nothing too firm. But I love having either side rubbed in a very steady rhythm. You'll know when you've got it, believe me."
> **Inara, 46, writer**

> "I like pressure a little above the clitoris, not right on it. Pressure should be firm and fairly steady, though changing in response to my own rhythm and signals (i.e., not the same no matter what, and not changing capriciously)."
> **Mae, 31, graduate student**

> "Light pinching/pulling, sometimes light pressure while circling. It's not a friggin' elevator button."
> **Seraphin, 40, technology strategist**

> "My clitoris can only be touched in a downward motion or a side-to-side motion. If you come up from the vagina over the clitoris, like toward my belly button, it's extremely uncomfortable and totally takes me out of the experience. It sets me back a good few steps."
> **Emily, 30, attorney**

Other women want you to offer them a combo platter:

> "It feels great to have my clitoris stimulated by fingers during intercourse, and that leads to greater orgasms with me."
> **Pearl, 22, chemist**

> "The best is light touching or licking of the clitoris while penetrating hard into the vagina with your fingers."
> **Heather, 25, executive assistant**

How do you like a man to touch your clitoris during foreplay?

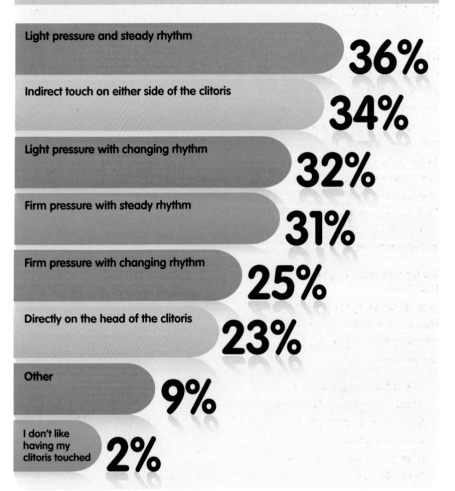

Light pressure and steady rhythm — **36%**

Indirect touch on either side of the clitoris — **34%**

Light pressure with changing rhythm — **32%**

Firm pressure with steady rhythm — **31%**

Firm pressure with changing rhythm — **25%**

Directly on the head of the clitoris — **23%**

Other — **9%**

I don't like having my clitoris touched — **2%**

Note: Respondents were allowed to select more than one answer to the question.

Other Great Ways to Use Your Hands

A woman's orgasm does not live by clit alone. We asked about all the other ways they like to be touched, and this is what they had to say about it:

Inara likes "pretty much everything," while 30-year-old artist Marla wants you to "take careful note of every surface of my body and love it as much as I do. The sheer act of loving ME makes all the difference." Paige recommends, "Constant pressure is good, anywhere, similar to a regular massage." Likewise, 40-year-old scientist Carrie has this advice: "Touch me all over my body: pinching, light scratching, tickling (early on only as part of playfully getting in the mood)." Here are some more specifics on how women want your nimble hands and fingers to go to work on the rest of their bodies:

> "Figure out where the tickle point is. If she likes to be tickled, fine, but otherwise, make sure you're touching her in a way that makes her moan instead of giggle."
> **Bryn, 41, secretary**

> "I like having my nipples pinched during sex."
> **Kate, 34, physician**

> "I love when they grab my hips, rub my breasts, tug my hair, USE THEM!"
> **Grape, 32, model/actress**

> "Learn how to stimulate the G-spot!"
> **Jennifer, 34, nonprofit worker**

One popular tourist destination didn't appear on our poll, but got special mention in several women's comments. But which one, you ask? Yes, it's the *gluteus maximus*. Several women in our survey say they want you to fondle, grab, squeeze, and play with their bottoms during foreplay. In fact, most women actually like you to play with their back door, "but are too shy to ask," claims Nana, a 37-year-old marketing manager.

Many women love to have their butts and anuses stroked, manipulated, and penetrated during intercourse as well. Ginger, a 38-year-old project manager, describes a technique of "rubbing the two halves of my buttocks and then pulling them apart-together-apart repeatedly" as being "very stimulating." Heather, 28, a travel photographer, loves it when her lover is "squeezing my butt, touching my clit, holding me right before I come." And Marla, 30, an artist, gave us this memorable motto: "Dick in the pink and pinky in the stink!"

It's okay. We're not sure how we feel about that last quotation either.

Besides clitoral stimulation, how else do you like to be physically stimulated?

Using his mouth and tongue on parts of my body (in addition to his fingers) **80%**

Playing with my nipples **70%**

Inserting one or more fingers into my vagina **69%**

Stroking my breasts **62%**

Stimulating my G-spot **52%**

Firm pressure of the entire palm against my pubic mound **51%**

Using something with a little bit of vibration (adult toy) **46%**

Stroking my pubic mound gently up and down **40%**

Using his fingers simultaneously on the vagina and anus **32%**

Other **5%**

1% I don't like my gentials touched

Note: Respondents were allowed to select more than one answer to the question.

Push My Buttons
(The Wrong Ways)

Some guys seem to be the ones who push all the *wrong* buttons. You know the type: He comes on too strong, moves too fast, and generally makes a woman feel like she's suddenly on the losing side of a WWE match. Or he does the exact opposite, leaving gals to wonder whether he's interested at all. Most mistakes fall under three broad categories of bad lovers.

Bad Lover No. 1: The Brute

Brutes can be aggressive or too impatient; they clumsily grope and paw their paramour, and lacking any gentleness or finesse, they can irritate or hurt their partners. Their crimes include:

GROPING

"Thick, hammy hands are a turnoff."
Shelley, 38, artist

"I'm not a piece of fruit to squeeze."
Sylvia, 48, marketing rep

"Groping clumsily. Use some finesse, guys."
Roxanne, 45, writer

You get the picture. Singled out for special mention in the groping category is misuse of the genitalia. Here are three big no-no's:

"Putting his finger inside the vagina too roughly."
Annabelle, age and occupation withheld

"Trying to force his whole hand inside my vagina."
Allison, age and occupation withheld

"Touching genitals too soon and/or too hard."
Andrea, 40, administrative manager

COMING ON TOO STRONG

"I hate when they use their hands roughly, or with too much pressure or speed," says Georgie, 43, an editor. She's not the only one. Although there is a time and a place for manhandling, generally the erogenous zones aren't included. Annie, a 62-year-old writer, doesn't like "too much pressure on the erogenous zones. My body is very sensitive and that would turn me off."

Too much pressure on the clitoris is a common complaint. Daisy, a 40-year-old stay-at-home mom, is not a fan of a man "rubbing it like there's a stain." In addition to applying too much pressure, "applying too many fingers at once" is also a turnoff, at least for Taylor, a 35-year-old teacher, as well as 42-year-old domestic executive Dawn, who dislikes "pushing a finger or fingers inside too hard."

The clitoris isn't the only scene of the crime when it comes to being too aggressive. Nana, a 37-year-old marketing executive, has a problem with a man "getting too forceful with his finger in my anus." And Elizabeth, a 28-year-old advertising sales manager, is equally annoyed by men "inserting too many fingers and playing with the nipples too long, until I feel numb."

Thirty-year-old Emily sums it up nicely when she tells us nothing turns her off more than a man "being too rough with my sensitive lady parts."

MOVING IN TOO FAST FOR THE KILL

Slow down, guys! Jumping straight for the erogenous zones before your partner is ready for you to go there is a big no-no. Remember what we (and our women) said about teasing? Heather, a 37-year-old marine biologist, asks that you "at least get your fingers wet first."

Here's what women said did *not* work for them:

> "Making the clitoris his first move. Touch any other part of my body first."
> **Keite, 31, office manager**

> "Sticking fingers into places without warning, or without sufficient lubrication."
> **Alina, 25, academic**

> "Sticking a finger in an orifice (vagina or anus) when it's not expected."
> **Pearl, 22, chemist**

> "Going straight for the clitoris with too-firm pressure, before properly 'heating the oven.'"
> **Summer, 27, TV advertising executive**

> "Dry insertion of anything."
> **Beth, 43, designer**

> "Going too fast right from the start. You have to work your way up to the faster speeds."
> **Stacey, 33, marketing professional**

Bottom line? "Men need to know that just sticking their fingers inside and jabbing away does not feel good," advises Dawn, a 29-year-old public relations executive. "Be gentle, go slow, take your time, and pay lots of attention to the clitoris first. That way I will be wet enough when you insert a finger and it will feel good."

Bad Lover No. 2: The Wimp

Just as being too rough and aggressive can blow it, so can going too far in the other direction. Women don't necessarily want "bad boys," but neither do they want someone who doesn't know when to be firm with his hands. According to our respondents, wimps are too timid, flimsy, and inconsistent when using their hands, buzzing all over the map like a mosquito but never giving their unsatisfied partners what they crave. "Quick and jerky, like a rabbit," notes Allison, a 34-year-old grant writer, about these disappointing characters. "They're all over the place," says Leslie, 30, a national account specialist. And Sally, a 35-year-old administrator, compares their "moving around too much" to having ADD. Other complaints:

> "No touching or hesitant, inconsistent touching."
> **Helena, 39, professor**

> "Tickling."
> **Denise, age and occupation withheld**

> "No more pressure than you'd give a peeled banana."
> **Vanessa, 35, administrator**

> "Acting timid."
> **Jennifer, 30, banking specialist**

> "Being 'fluttery.'"
> **Rachel, 45, entrepreneur**

> "Doing nothing with their hands, or giving me friendly pats and massages with them. Not sexy."
> **Bryn, 41, secretary**

Overwhelmingly, however, the women taking our survey complained that the most unforgivable thing that the Wimp does with his hands is . . . "nothing" (Breanna, 51, publishing executive); "not touching me enough—everywhere" (Brianna, 30, marketing specialist); "going on autopilot" (Inara, 46, writer); and "not doing anything with them" (Heather, 28, travel photographer). When we asked Z.B., 27, what she wishes guys wouldn't do, her answer was one word: "Stop."

Bad Lover No. 3: The Clod

Clods are clueless. Their handiwork is all thumbs: They're oblivious to the signals she's putting out, they don't think about what they are doing, and (sin of sins) they lack imagination. They can be inconsiderate and are capable of making truly stupid mistakes. Here are some of the many ways you can recognize one, and hopefully avoid being labeled a Clod:

> "Fumbling around, not knowing where he is."
> **Beth, 43, designer**

> "Overstimulating the clit and/or not paying attention to my cues."
> **Caroline, 29, teacher**

> "Going immediately to the breasts/nipples and just staying there. BORING!"
> **Michelle, 35, marketing project manager**

> "Being too technical. Like he has to do it and be over with it to get inside me."
> **Matilda, 32, pharmacist**

> "Wrong touch, wrong pressure, wrong time. Or does something he thinks I love when I've made it clear I don't."
> **Alex, 35, college professor**

One clod maneuver in particular that doesn't sit well with our respondents is described by Mae, a 31-year-old graduate student: "Putting fingers in the anus and then into the vagina. This goes for other objects as well. Much as I like having to visit the gynecologist later to get rid of the resulting infection." Twenty-nine-year-old lawyer Troy asks that you "just don't switch back and forth between vagina and anus with the same fingers." And 32-year-old model/actress Grape, 32, like, totally agrees: "Think it's cool to stick it in the anus and then the vajayjay afterwards . . . like, hello? Germs don't mix well that way."

Top Hand Techniques

While we're on the subject of hands—and on a more positive note—let's talk about what kind of touch *does* work. Every woman remembers fondly the man whose hands sent her over the moon, leaving her gasping for more. It's the kind of memory that fuels her hottest solo sessions—it's maybe even what she fantasizes about during lovemaking. Scan the amazing hand techniques in this section and see which one you might make your own signature move.

G Marks the Spot

"Without a doubt, having my G-spot stimulated with his hand—AMAZING," raves Jennifer, 34, a nonprofit worker. Researchers debate just what the G-spot is; some say it is the female equivalent of the prostate; others claim that it is simply the tail end of the clitoris. But you only need to worry about where it is on your partner and how to make it sing. Thirty-year-old household engineer Arianna tells you how to find it: "With one finger inside, move it as if to say 'come here,' and it hits the right spot." It's a ridged, rippled area about the size of a quarter, on the inside front wall. Because it's made from erectile tissue, it will swell up when you stimulate it. Here are some tips from women on how to do just that:

"Both fingers in and sort of scissor-kicking them quickly. Sort of like 'let your fingers do the walking,' but they're speed-walking or maybe dancing, doing the Twist a bit." **Seraphin, 40, technology strategist**

"Fingers on the G-spot and clit at the same time."
Nara, 41, massage therapist

"G-spot stimulation with two or more fingers."
Suzy, 32, business executive

"Rubbing the G-spot with your finger while giving oral."
Roxy, 31, administrator

"Rubbing the pubic mound while stimulating the G-spot with their thumb."
Ava, age and occupation withheld

Let Your Fingers Do the Walking

As great as the G-spot is, there are plenty of other fun things women would like you to do with your hands. Troy shares this experience with us: "A long-fingered man explored my vagina very thoroughly, finding spots I'd never felt probed before, while looking into my eyes. Extremely sexy, very intimate, I felt completely exposed." Alina, a 25-year-old academic, likes "gentle teasing to the point of orgasm, and then applying direct pressure and pinching my clit."

"My boyfriend in college could vibrate his fingers superfast, like a vibrator," says Sara, a 27-year-old CPA. "Amazing."

Other techniques that send women into ecstasy? Try these:

> "Combining clitoral stimulation with occasional finger penetration."
> **Allison, age and occupation withheld**

> "Two fingers in and out very fast."
> **Zelda, 26, actress**

> "Three fingers over the clitoris like strumming a guitar."
> **Sasha, 44, business executive**

> "I can't say it's the most 'amazing,' but one of the fastest ways to give me an orgasm is by applying firm pressure to my clitoris and then rubbing the finger back and forth in that perfect rhythm we all have."
> **Adrienne, 33, graduate student**

> "Perfect pressure to give me a clitoral orgasm, starting slow and ending fast with increasing amounts of pressure from start to finish."
> **Elizabeth, 28, advertising sales manager**

> "His whole hand under me, slightly lifting me up while rubbing everything and fingers entering every so often!"
> **Paige, age and occupation withheld**

> "He listened to my cues and believed me when I said that only on the spot really worked."
> **Alex, 33 college professor**

> "As we were kissing, he put his middle and ring finger in my vagina. I wasn't lubricated at all, so it seemed awfully coarse at the time. He left them there, just pressing them up into me, while he kissed me and touched my neck and my breasts. Then as I was getting wet, he started moving his fingers in and out. The backwardness of it was a little rough and aggressive, but it felt amazing."
> **Bryn, 41, secretary**

Serve Up a Combo Platter

If your fingers are good, just imagine what you can do using your fingers *and* your tongue. These women certainly are:

> "Fingers in my vagina while performing oral sex."
> **Richelle, 47, attorney**

> "Using his hands (e.g., inserting one or more fingers into my vagina) while performing oral sex—what a great combination! Also doing this while making out—what a turn-on!"
> **Sunny, 36, project manager**

> "Combination of oral sex and fingers on clitoris and inside."
> **Sarah, 47, attorney**

> "Using his mouth and tongue on parts of my body while stroking my inner thighs. Or cupping my butt and lifting me to his mouth."
> **Sylvia, 48, marketing rep**

The "Six Pack"

What else can you do? Try what Abbey, a 30-year-old designer, calls "the 'Six Pack.' The shocker. In other words, simultaneous vaginal and anal insertion." She's not the only one who likes it:

> "Two fingers in my vagina and one rubbing my anus. I think there were also fingers on my clitoris. There were fingers everywhere!"
> **Carrie, 40, scientist**

> "Vagina and anus together. I don't know exactly what he did, but it was amazing."
> **Jenny, 28, medical office manager**

> "One hand with a finger in the vagina and anus. The other hand with finger or tongue on clitoris."
> **Nana, 37, marketing manager**

> "Using his fingers on both clit and anus, while applying a firm pressure on my pubic mound."
> **Pat, 56, project manager**

> "What I lovingly refer to as 'the Six-Pack' . . . thumb and middle finger in the vagina and anus, respectively, when coming from behind. Whew."
> **Ulla, 29, performer**

> "Having one finger in my anus, two in my vagina, and stimulating my clitoris at the same time . . . I had an orgasm almost instantly."
> **Heather, 37, marine biologist**

Coming from Behind

As any real estate agent will tell you, location is everything. There's something primal about being taken from behind, whether it's full-on intercourse or manual manipulation. Here are a few things you can do when you're going at it from the back:

> "Standing behind me while inserting his fingers into my vagina. His hand/wrist was stimulating my clitoris at the same time because of our body position."
> **Pearl, 22, chemist**

> "He had me face down and was taking me from behind, using his hand on and around my clitoris at the same time."
> **Inara, 46, writer**

> "His left arm around my back so he could insert his fingers in my vagina, from behind, while his right hand stimulated my clitoris on top."
> **Helen, 48, executive**

> "I like it when a guy uses his fingers on my clitoris when we're doing doggy style. That's probably my favorite position/ technique."
> **Emily, 30, attorney**

Don't Forget the Total Package

It's not just all about the quivering loins and trembling thighs. Don't neglect the rest of her body; she'll thank you for it. Helena, a 39-year-old professor, sighs, "I always remember the men who had just the most amazing touch all over my body. You totally lose yourself and your mind and all real awareness of where exactly it is that they might be touching you. I can have an orgasm from men who are super adept at this all-over-the-body technique." A few other choice experiences women would like to repeat:

> "Stroking my entire torso slowly while having intercourse, exploring and enjoying my body. It makes me feel sexy."
> **Frankie, 36, swim instructor**

> "Touching me everywhere but the clitoris for a bit . . . then making one slow and soft stroke over it."
> **Summer, 27, TV advertising executive**

> "Slow, soft strokes down the length of my body, with absolutely no rush. He seemed to be savoring the touch even more than I was, and it went on and on and on until I couldn't take it anymore and had to have him inside me."
> **Michelle, 35, marketing project manager**

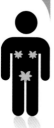

"He listened to my cues and believed me when I said that only on the spot really worked."

Alex, 33 college professor

Let Your Fingers Do the Talking

We couldn't have a chapter about hands without talking about masturbation. We know men like to watch women pleasure themselves. (In Cynthia's book *What Men Really Want in Bed*, 82 percent said they like to see a woman masturbate—and not a single man said he didn't.) But how does it make women feel to be observed?

Although the majority of women say they're comfortable putting on a bit of a show when it comes to masturbation, like so many topics on our sex survey, the most common answer is: *It depends.*

"It totally depends on how comfortable I am with the person," notes Annette. "With some people it's fun, but with others I am self-conscious." Designer Sophie, 45, says, "It depends. If he's participating a little, touching and getting into it, that's great, but

How do you feel about a man watching you masturbate?

I like it—it turns me on and he can see what I like **37%**

I don't like it—it makes me feel self-conscious **26%**

I don't mind, but it doesn't do anything for me **23%**

Other **14%**

Note: Percentages may not equal 100% due to rounding.

not if he's just passively watching." Bryn, a 41-year-old secretary, tells us that she hasn't ever tried it, "but I wouldn't be averse to it. Might be educational for him."

Others are less enthusiastic about the prospect of starring in a private show:

> "I've never really been good at masturbating, so I feel like I'd have to kind of pretend."
> **Camilla, 25, advertising manager**

> "I am one of those few lame women who can't masturbate. It's sad but true. I bought books, I tried. It doesn't work. I can't fake it."
> **Seraphin, 40, technology strategist**

> "I can't do it effectively if a man is watching—at least, this is something I'm convinced of, so I've always declined to let men watch. I get very much into my own fantasy world and having a man there watching would be too much of a distraction."
> **Mae, 31, graduate student**

So if you do want to see how she pleasures herself—either because you want to learn something or it just plain turns you on—make sure she knows how much you like it. Do what you can to put her at ease. Put your hand over hers and guide it to her clitoris. Whisper in her ear that you'd love to watch her masturbate. If and when she climaxes, tell her how beautiful and hot her orgasm was to watch. Whatever you do, don't pressure her. If she doesn't want to touch herself in front of you, let it go.

What about when the shoe is on the other foot, so to speak? Over half the women we surveyed like the idea of watching their man masturbate. In fact, singer Heather, 31, shouts "LOVE IT!" But of course, for most women, it depends—on the man, or her mood, or other factors. For Annette, "it depends on how comfortable I am with him. And I like to be part of the action, licking or touching other areas while watching him do himself." Rachel, 45, an entrepreneur, says it "depends on the man and how he's doing it. As performance, it's fascinating."

Seraphin expands on the topic for us: "Sometimes it's erotic. It depends on the guy, how he masturbates, and how often. This one guy I dated had this monster dildo he shoved up his ass while whacking off. NOT erotic. And then he wondered why I couldn't marry him."

Other women are not as traumatized, but simply haven't gotten around to it yet. Lawyer Sheba, 35, is a bit reticent. "I like the idea of it, but it's not something that he has ever done, and I'm not comfortable asking for it." Meanwhile, Marla, a 30-year-old artist, says, "I don't think I would mind. Just don't let me walk in and be surprised . . . WEIRD."

Still other respondents have their reasons for not wanting to watch their men pleasure themselves. Thirty-five-year-old Karen, a student, says, "I'd prefer he not service himself. I'm turned on knowing he has the self-control to wait for me to satisfy him." (What she doesn't know is that many men masturbate simply for stress release.) Ginger admits, "I like watching anyone enjoy themselves, but I'm greedy and wouldn't want to miss out on the opportunity for something for myself, too." Of course, if you see what he likes and can duplicate it, and vice versa, there will be more than enough for everyone!

How do you feel about watching a man masturbate?

I like it—it gives me ideas and turns me on **50%**

No thanks—let him do it on his own time **23%**

I don't mind, but it doesn't do anything for me **20%**

Other **9%**

Note: *Percentages may not equal 100% due to rounding.*

Chapter 4

Oral Sex: The Good, the Bad, and the Ugly

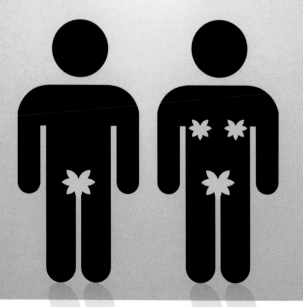

Guys, we know that you love oral sex—getting it *and* giving it. In case you need a statistic with which to reassure her, more than 80 percent of the guys surveyed for Cynthia's book *What Men Really Want in Bed* say they love lavishing oral attention on their gal's privates. But many men are hesitant to go south on a woman for fear of doing it "wrong" or worries that she doesn't really like it.

Well, fear not. Like you, the vast majority of women adore being the recipient of oral sex. Your tongue can deliver just the right amount of pressure and speed to send her into the stratosphere, as long as you pay attention to her cues. So it pays to become a cunnilingus expert, especially where your particular recipient is concerned. Your gal may not want or need it every single time you get busy, but it's a rare woman who doesn't care for it at all. And in that case, don't sweat it. "If we say we don't like it, believe us. Don't take it personally; it's just not our thing," counsels Cari, a 26-year-old administrative assistant.

So what *did* they say? Read on.

What Women Wish Men Knew about Oral Sex

Yeah, we'll say it again: Every woman is different, and that's especially true when it comes to oral sex. Some gals may like full-on contact with your tongue; others may want you to circle their love button. One woman may need a light touch, while another may truly want you to eat her out. You'll only know through trial and error (and don't be afraid to ask for directions).

But there are a few common themes when it comes to women and oral sex. We figured that if we shared some of them with you, you'd have a head start. Pun intended.

We Like It. We Really, Really Like It.

Let's get it right out into the open: Women love oral sex. "It's just as good for us as it is when we do it to them," says Sarah, a 31-year-old health-care professional. And they want you to do it more, more, more—as often as possible, in fact. Dawn, a 29-year-old PR executive, claims "it should be incorporated every time we have sex," while 39-year-old Jane, a businesswoman, suggests, "Just do it all the time!" (Don't worry. We know you're not machines.)

But know that a woman's preferences regarding oral sex are as individual as she is. For example, Helena, a 39-year-old professor, says, "I like oral sex, but it isn't a must-have all the time for me. I would also sometimes like a man to combine it with inserting

> **"If it's done with passion and they're enjoying it, then it's probably good."**
>
> **Paige, age and occupation withheld**

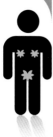

something inside me. And for guys who are 'into' oral sex, just make sure your partner is on board with you wanting to dive down there for long periods of time! I like lots of other things, too."

And, while we saw in chapter 3 that many women love oral sex as part of foreplay, others consider it the main event. "I want it to last longer," says Carrie, a 40-year-old scientist, "not just long enough to get me aroused so he can move on to intercourse. Don't use it as a means to an end." The moral of the story? Even if your gal loves mouth music as a prelude to lovemaking, every once in a while, make it the featured—and only—piece on the playlist.

Show Some Enthusiasm, Please

When a woman lets you go down on her, she's expressing a great deal of trust. So for most of our respondents, it's important that you show a little passion for the endeavor. Moan, sigh, make eye contact, or tell her how good she feels and tastes. Otherwise, she may have trouble relaxing and enjoying herself—because she'll be worrying about you. (For better or worse, most women have been brought up to be people-pleasers, even in bed.) "I need him to convey total enthusiasm for it," says Abbey, a 30-year-old designer. She, like many other women, would prefer that you actually enjoy oral sex and don't just see it as a means to getting her off—in part so they can relax and get into it.

"I find it's a very personal, caring thing for a guy to do," says Camilla, a 25-year-old advertising manager. "It shows me he likes me and my body. So as long as he's enjoying himself and not rushing through it, I'll be very happy."

In fact, enthusiasm even trumps technique—and leads to a better experience for everyone. "If it's done with passion and they're enjoying it, then it's probably good," says Paige. Adds Michelle, a 35-year-old marketing project manager, "If he expresses that he loves it and is in no hurry, I can relax and really enjoy it."

And if you *don't* like performing oral sex on her, don't do it out of obligation. That's the last thing women want. "I'd rather be doing something we both enjoy," says 45-year-old Karren, an attorney, while 29-year-old Heather, a pastry chef, says, "If you're not enjoying yourself, I'd rather you just stop than pretend."

Remember, women are extremely intuitive, so the chances are good she'll pick up on your distaste. "If you don't really, truly, deep down love it, I'm going to be able to tell, and it will make me feel like you're doing a chore, rather than something you love," says Pat, a 56-year-old project manager. Adds Taylor, a 65-year-old comedy writer, "It's not a job that requires sacrifice!"

One reason women need reassurance is that many of us have had less-than-stellar experiences. "You've gotta convince me that you love it," says Caroline, a 29-year-old teacher. "A guy once made the mistake of letting me know he didn't like doing it, and that killed our sexual relationship. How could I enjoy what he was doing if I knew he didn't like doing it in the first place?"

So don't be shy. If you love giving her oral sex, let her know! And if you don't, mum's the word, especially if you're hoping to get the same treatment. "They need to at least pretend to like it if they want reciprocation," says Kate, a 35-year-old writer.

Listen to Her Cues

You may think that you've got the world's best oral sex technique. And that may be true, but it won't do you any good if it doesn't work for your current partner. That's why we can't overstress the importance of paying attention to her feedback. Listen to her cues: her moans, her sighs, her squirms, her expressions of delight—or the lack of them—to figure out what's working, and what's not.

Communication Is Key

Yes, we know we've probably beaten this one into your brain by now, but if you take just one thing away from this book (and we hope you'll take more!), it's that good communication can make or break it when it comes to sharing a mutually satisfying sexual encounter. Although you don't want to analyze things to death, having an idea of what turns your partner on before you hit the bedroom and then using that knowledge is not only going to be more fun for both of you, but it will also increase the odds of a repeat experience.

> "Discussing likes and dislikes beforehand is a plus! I'd like to know what your turn-ons and -offs are, just as much as I would like you to know mine. Communication is the key!"
> **Cari, 26, administrative assistant**

> "If you're comfortable with your partner, the sky's the limit about what you're willing to try. Keep communication open and don't be selfish; try to make her happy, and she'll try to make you happy."
> **Annette, 44, manager**

> "Good sex is usually the product of either a) chemistry or b) good communication. If you don't have chemistry, you really have to work on the communication."
> **Bryn, 41, secretary**

Here's more advice from our survey respondents:

"We are very sensitive down there. Maybe your last girlfriend liked it rough, but every girl is different, and you have to pay attention to our cues on how we like it."
Heather, 25, executive assistant

"Listen to my nonverbal responses, and wait for the 'right' time to go down there. I need to be appropriately aroused beforehand. If they think it's going to be a case of going down straightaway and that's going to do the trick, then they're mistaken!"
Allison, age and occupation withheld

"The biggest mistake he can make is when he tries to create his own rhythm by going faster and slower and faster, rather than responding to my rhythm and signals."
Mae, 31, graduate student

"It's not rocket science. It should be obvious what is pleasurable or not from my response. If one of us isn't into it, it's not worthwhile."
Maureen, 45, archeologist

"Adjust to nonverbal cues. It can be stimulating, but it won't always lead to orgasm, so know when to move on."
Alison, 36, homemaker

"Listen to our rhythmic responses."
Helen, 48, executive

"If my verbal cues indicate that I'm enjoying something, *don't stop doing that.*"
Ellen, 37, Web development team manager

When in Doubt, Ask for Directions

This brings us to our next tip. Although nonverbal cues are a great way to gauge your woman's arousal level, it never hurts to simply ask her for feedback—or even instructions. Every woman is different, so you have to discover what works for her specifically, because what worked for your ex may not work for her. "There are many ways to perform oral sex, but not all ways are preferred by all women," says Denise. "Find out what she likes by asking her." (Most of us understand that you don't have ESP.)

Another reason to speak up is that she may be reticent to give you instructions. "I'm not necessarily going to say what I like," says Z.B., a 27-year-old researcher. What's more, they appreciate being asked: "Do NOT be shy," advises Roxie, a 39-year-old communications professional. "Ask the lady what she likes—that's hot."

Of course, if you do ask her for input, *listen to her answer.* Nothing will frustrate a woman faster than feeling like she's not being heard. "I tell guys what I wish they knew," says Seraphin, a 40-year-old technology strategist, "but I just wish they would remember so I don't have to repeat myself. It's annoying and unnerving and uncomfortable. Why is it they remember so much stupid, useless trivia and can't remember the important stuff?" Says an exasperated Heather, a 28-year-old travel photographer: "If they would just stay down and follow my directions, I would come."

Be Gentle

When asked "What is the one thing you wish men knew about oral sex?" many women responded with a plea for gentleness down below. "My clitoris is very sensitive, and I don't like a lot of direct pressure—it's just too much," says Inara, 46, echoing the feeling of many survey takers. Consistent, light pressure seems to be the way to go with several (although not all) gals.

And you should definitely ease off after her orgasm. "After I come, it's too sensitive for a few moments to keep going," says Murphy, a 60-year-old artist. "Just give me a break and then I will come for you again!"

Use Your Fingers

Many women like you to boost their pleasure by combining oral action with deft finger work. "Fingers can enhance the experience," says Katia, a 34-year-old financial executive. For some women, it's more than an enhancement: It's downright necessary. "Tongue is nice, but it doesn't take me all the way," says Sara, a 27-year-old CPA. "Hands and fingers are needed, too."

You can use your fingers and hands in a variety of ways. Stroke her skin, play with her nipples, give your tongue a break and massage her clitoris with a finger or two. She may even want you to slip a finger inside her. "Penetration with a finger while licking my clitoris is great!" exclaims Liz, a 36-year-old physician.

However, this is one technique you should definitely approach slowly and carefully. Caress her with your hands, slide a finger gently inside her, but do *not* under any circumstances jab her with your fingers. "There's no gold up in there—*quit digging your finger up into me*!" exclaims Caroline. "One is enough, and just to feel it there or slowly moving in and out is a great addition to what your tongue is doing to my clit, but when you start jamming around up in there, it pisses me off. It's completely unnecessary!"

Find the Clitoris

More than one woman in our survey avoided offering specific advice on technique. Instead, they advised men to simply find the one organ in a woman's body whose sole purpose is sexual pleasure. "You know that thing called the clitoris?" asks Carrie, a 28-year-old entrepreneur. "Well, find it, dammit! Then play with it!"

And here's *how* to find it, for you men who—due to inexperience or other circumstances—might not know. (Don't be embarrassed. Everyone has to start somewhere.) At the top of her pubic area, where the folds of her skin (her labia) meet, there's a little hard nub covered by a hood of skin. If you were to pull back that hood, you'd see the clitoral glans, which, by the way, is usually way too sensitive for a full frontal assault. Because every woman's clitoris is different, it never hurts to ask her to guide your hand to the right place. Chances are she'd be delighted by your interest.

Variety Is the Spice of Life

One of the most frequent bits of advice our survey takers gave about oral sex was to mix up your mouth moves, and pay close attention to her responses. Your woman isn't necessarily going to like the same technique each time. "What feels best changes, so your technique should change, too," says Maren, a 32-year-old physical therapist. "It's important to use different speeds and try different things," advises Blair, a 27-year-old lawyer. "Don't just go really slow or really fast. Make sure there's variety." And, as we said previously, she isn't necessarily going to like the same move your ex did.

However, the time to *stop* varying your moves is when it's clear she likes what you're doing—or when she's racing toward orgasm. At that point, changing position, technique, or pressure may distract her. "Find something that works, and stick with it," says Kristy, a 34-year-old pharmacist. "Don't change every two minutes."

Remember that her entire genital area will respond to your attention. "Explore and don't just stay in one spot, a.k.a. the clitoris," says 20-year-old Kyleranne, a student. Forty-four-year-old manager Annette offers specific instructions: "Kiss her *everywhere*, not just the clitoris. Suck the labia (both sides), put your tongue in her, nibble. Make out with her down there!"

Another key skill: multitasking. Use your hands to augment what your mouth is doing. Touch and stroke her entire body. Kiss her inner thighs. Play with her breasts and, even better, her nipples. "I love having my nipples played with while we are having sex of any kind," says Casi.

It's Not a Race to the Finish— Take Your Time

Patience, grasshopper. Oral sex is an art that can't be rushed—that's the consensus of the women in our survey. For best results, start slow, take your time, and build up steam. "You're going to need to be there for a while, so stamina is crucial," says Keite, a 31-year-old office manager. "Don't go in there full-throttle or you won't make it."

Other comments and advice from our respondents:

"Kiss my belly and inner thighs first, build up the suspense and my desire before you actually get to my genitals. Make me want you really badly before you actually get there."
Andrea, 40, administrative manager

"I need to take my time and can't be rushed."

Georgie, 43, editor

"Take the time to figure out what makes me tick. We're all different, and like different things."

Adrienne, 33, graduate student

"It takes a while . . . don't stop so much. Consistency on the clitoris. It's okay to use your finger to stimulate if you need a break. Just don't stop."

Nana, 37, marketing manager

"Slow down. It should be like making out, not frantic."

Sam, 35, lawyer

"It takes more than two minutes, so vary your speed and pressure. I hate being licked up and down. It feels like a tongue bath."

Vanessa, 35, administrator

"Start slow, and then get faster as she gets into it. Lighter pressure on the clitoris."

Suzy, 32, business executive

"Take your time . . . it would be nice if they enjoyed it and did not treat it like a juicy burger they did not know what to do with."

Marla, 30, artist

"Slow and steady. Patience. Let me build up to orgasm without too much expectation. I need to know he enjoys it."

Beth, 43, designer

To sum up? Listen to the advice of Elizabeth, the 28-year-old advertising sales manager, whose comment encapsulates everything we heard: "Explore the entire vagina inside out. Cover lots of surface area of genital skin. I need to be warmed up! You can't go to town right away. Start slow and soft, then build up speed and pressure the more I get excited. Zone in on the clit once I'm there and ready to orgasm. Then keep the rhythm consistent (fast!)."

Go Out of Your Way to Make Her Feel Comfortable

Thanks to the barrage of marketing for so-called douches, feminine deodorant, and the like, many women feel self-conscious about how they smell "down there." It's a shame, because not only are these products not necessary—the vagina is basically a self-cleaning organ, and douching upsets the balance—but most men like a woman's natural scent. To put her at ease, perform your mouth music with gusto, and, as 29-year-old Troy advises, "always reassure the woman about her smell and taste and tell her you like it. A lot of women worry about it."

Whatever you do, heed the words of Jyllian, a 44-year-old engineer and mother: "Oh good lord, please NEVER EVER make a comment about the smell or taste. NEVER EVER."

Enough said.

Remember, It's Just the Appetizer

Yes, many women do consider oral sex as just that—sex—and it can certainly be the main event in a lovemaking session. Yet several women in our survey remind you that it's often "just the appetizer," as Paula, 55, puts it, whether or not they've had an orgasm. In fact, going on too long can backfire, and here's why:

> "Once I've come, I want to move on to penetration . . . NOW."
> **Daisy, 40, stay-at-home mom**

> "I love oral sex, but almost never come from it, and that doesn't have to be the point. It definitely gets me fired up for penile penetration."
> **Scarlet, 34, chef**

> "As part of sex, it is great, yet nothing replaces actual intercourse. Don't feel pressured to perform oral sex for a long time."
> **Monica, 49, restaurant owner**

> "I get self-conscious. I don't like to feel pressured to have an orgasm. I can and will, but if that is the only outcome he is looking for, I feel too pressured and can't relax enough to let go."
> **Elizabeth, 32, mental health provider**

Keep in mind that her pleasure may be affected by factors totally beyond your control. "If I've had anything alcoholic to drink, I'm probably not going to climax from oral sex," says Roxanne, a 45-year-old writer.

So don't put too much pressure on yourself or your partner. Enjoy giving her pleasure, but get Zen about it and let go of the outcome. "I think there's too much pressure for men to bring me to an orgasm," says Camilla, 25, an advertising manager. "I love receiving oral sex for the entire experience. It's not all about the ending."

And Sometimes We Don't Want Appetizers

Yes, you can have too much of a good thing. Oral sex isn't something she's going to expect you—or want you—to perform every time, according to our survey respondents. "I don't always want it, and when I say stop, stop," says Julie, a 43-year-old artist and writer. And don't worry: She'll still enjoy sex.

Trust her when she says she's not in the mood for you going down on her. "If my head is in the wrong place you might as well be sucking on my elbow for all the good it's doing me," says Jackie, a 50-year-old artist. Whatever you do, don't take it personally.

What's the Biggest Mistake Men Make During Oral Sex?

Wondering how you can avoid committing an oral faux pas? For one, don't stage a full-frontal assault on her bean. By far the biggest mistake men make when performing oral sex on a woman is applying too much direct pressure on the clitoris, too soon. Although many women like and need pressure on the hood that covers the clitoral glans, nearly 33 percent said they can't stand it when their partner uses his tongue like he's trying to remove a stain from the carpet. Her clitoris can't take direct scrubbing, guys.

Next mistake, and we can't say this often enough: Women want to know that you like going down on them. "I think the biggest mistake is doing oral sex because it's 'expected,' not because he enjoys it and the pleasure it gives," says Sylvia, a 48-year-old marketing representative. "Like he's ticking off a list what must be done to get to intercourse. Did the neck, check; boobs, check . . ."

> **"I think the biggest mistake is doing oral sex because it's 'expected,' not because he enjoys it and the pleasure it gives."**
>
> **Sylvia, 48, marketing representative**

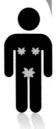

What's the biggest mistake men make when performing oral sex?

- Too much direct pressure on clitoris — **33%**
- He doesn't seem to be enjoying himself — **12%**
- Not enough attention to the clitoris — **12%**
- Not enough pressure — **8%**
- Other — **8%**
- Inconsistent rhythm — **8%**
- All of the above — **5%**
- I can feel his teeth — **4%**
- Trying to perform it in the first place—I don't like it — **3%**
- He doesn't listen when I tell him what I like — **3%**
- Lack of eye contact — **2%**
- Too slow — **1%**

Note: Percentages may not equal 100% due to rounding.

Finding the Best Rhythm and Pressure

We've touched on the subject of rhythm and pressure. Given the caveat that every woman is different, we found that a solid 50 percent of the women who took our survey want a combination of speeds and pressures. That does *not* mean, however, that you should be constantly speeding up and slowing down, or pretend like you're sending Morse code with your tongue. Most women said they like you to start with slow, light, teasing pressure that gradually builds in speed and intensity to send them over the edge. "Keep it steady," says 50-year-old Erika, a writer and teacher. Meanwhile, Beth says she needs side-to-side rhythmic stroking but "don't get messy all over the place and for God's sake don't stop."

Here again is an area where it's important to see what feedback her responses give you. "I need it to start slow and gentle, but I won't reach orgasm if it stays that way," says Keite, a 31-year-old office manager, "so it's important that he listen to my cues (or better yet, is totally in tune with how I feel)."

Which begs the question, how do you find out which rhythm and pressure *your* partner likes? Most women—45 percent in our survey—suggest that you watch their bodies and reactions closely. "Physically, it's pretty obvious what we like and don't like," says Grape, a 32-year-old model and actress. "That squirming like she's trying to get away?

That's because she is. Go easy. Most women will use their hips and pull your hair to get you on the right track." And don't worry: Most of the women we surveyed understand that it will take you a little while to get into the groove of what they like.

And if you're in doubt, 30 percent want you to just ask them what they like. Some women will be proactive and give you direct instructions, but many feel shy and worried about sounding like a drill sergeant. "It's helpful for the man to suggest, 'Say YES when you really like something so I'll know what's really working for you,'" says Roxie, the 39-year-old communications professional. "That way, the woman feels more comfortable about giving 'direction' or saying what she wants."

Roxie also offered a great suggestion: Make a game out of it. "Tell her, 'I'm going to try all sorts of different things and you're going to tell me when I'm getting warmer or colder—and when I'm getting HOT!'"

Remember, asking what she likes is different from *grilling* her. "I don't like to feel like I'm filling out a survey during the first few rounds," says Ginger, a 38-year-old project manager, "but I'm happy to answer questions if he's got lingering doubts."

You shouldn't feel shy about asking for direction, or embarrassed when she gives it to you. "Most guys go too fast and too light," says Mae. "Maybe it's just that I operate a bit different from most women, but I almost *always* have to instruct him on what to do."

What type of rhythm and pressure do you like during oral sex?

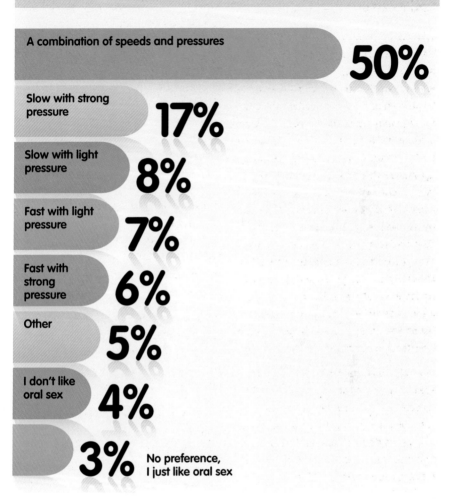

A combination of speeds and pressures — **50%**

Slow with strong pressure — **17%**

Slow with light pressure — **8%**

Fast with light pressure — **7%**

Fast with strong pressure — **6%**

Other — **5%**

I don't like oral sex — **4%**

3% No preference, I just like oral sex

Note: Percentages may not equal 100% due to rounding.

Here's the good news: Women are open to letting you do a bit of experimentation. "I like to see what a guy has to offer before I start offering suggestions or preferences," says Inara, a 46-year-old writer. "If he's hurting me (too much direct pressure), I'll let him know." Vicky, a 43-year-old professional water-skier, agrees: "You never know what skills he might have that I don't know about."

What's the best way for a man to find out what kind of oral sex you enjoy?

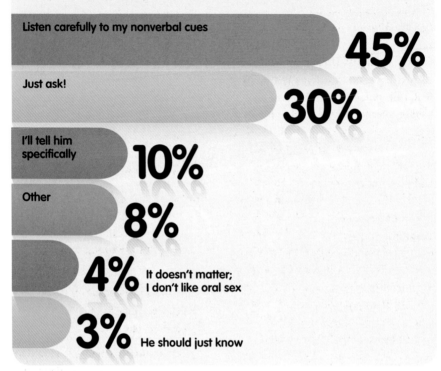

Listen carefully to my nonverbal cues
45%

Just ask!
30%

I'll tell him specifically
10%

Other
8%

4% It doesn't matter; I don't like oral sex

3% He should just know

Note: Percentages may not equal 100% due to rounding.

The Sexiest Thing to Do with Your Mouth

Despite what you might think from watching *Sex and the City* (and yes, we know, you only watched it because your girlfriend was and you had nothing else to do), most women don't talk with their friends in explicit detail about their sex lives. Oh, sure, we can be plenty snarky when recounting the gory details of a bad date who hunched over his Black-Berry the entire evening or who snapped at the waiter. And every woman has had to endure a girlfriend's cringe-inducing tale of the Man Who Is The One. But ask us about the sex, and we clam up. Well, your authors think this is a shame. You don't have to blog about your exploits, but let's give a shout-out to the dudes who do it right. So we asked women to name the most mind-blowing oral technique a partner had ever used on them. Here are the moves that put men in the Cunnilingus Hall of Fame.

He Sucked (But in a Good Way)

You know how it feels when you're inside her, surrounded by her warmth and wetness, and she clenches around you as you thrust? Or how insanely turned on you get during a really good blow job? Well, imagine doing something similar to her clitoris, which is, after all, composed of erectile tissue just like your member. Over and over, women cite a gentle sucking technique as a move that sends them into orbit:

"He used a combination of swirling his tongue around my clit and sucking on it with varying degrees of pressure."
Alina, 25, academic

"He sucked on my clit, while flicking his tongue back and forth across it."
Andrea, 40, administrative manager

"He sucked on my clitoris and then performed a slightly round tongue movement on it. I almost went unconscious."
Matilda, 32, pharmacist

"He sucked with his whole mouth around my clit and the surrounding area. He also breathed hotly on my clitoral area."
Heather, 25, executive assistant

"Swirling the tongue on the clit in circles and sucking at the same time, gently and then more forcefully."
Roxy, 31, administrator

"After I was already aroused, he moved his tongue around my clit several times and then sucked lightly on it."
Michelle, 36, management consultant

"I love soft licking followed by a surprising sucking."
Ava, age and occupation withheld

He Had a Magical Tongue

The bad news: There's no one oral technique that will work for every woman. The good news: There's no one oral technique that will work for every woman. This frees you to try anything and everything in your quest to send her over the edge. But where are you going to get good ideas that really work? (Hint: It's not the Internet.) Check out some real-life stories of how some men turned their tongues into finely honed instruments of pleasure:

"He drew the letters of the alphabet with his tongue on my clitoris."
Kelly, 32, wildlife biologist

"He had a really strong tongue—and he really seemed to like doing it."
Roxanne, 45, writer

"He had a tongue like a vibrator."
Shelley, 38, artist

"He put me on the dining room table after dinner and licked me in long strokes until I came."
Karren, 45, attorney

"A combination of suck, blow on the wet spot, lick (long and slow), then repeat!"
Pat, 56, project manager

"Slow, gentle, and deep tongue, like he was making out with my vag. Amazing."
Lulu, 35, defense attorney

"He penetrated me with his tongue."
Kyleranne, 20, student

"He used soft pressure with his tongue that slowly got harder . . . but not too hard!"
Marie, 26, teacher

"He did a little bit of everything all over: nibbling, sucking, long licks, short licks, sideways."
Georgie, 43, editor

"His tongue made circles around my clitoris"
Sasha, 44, business executive

"He had full mouth coverage with a strong sweep of the tongue, landing on the clit, releasing with a gentle suck. The movement across the vulva was tickled by day-old stubble. Bonus WOW."
Roxie, 35, communications professional

"He started really slow with long pressured strokes up and down around my labia, covering a lot of surface area across all of my genitals. I got superexcited, so when he finally came up to my clit I was almost already having an orgasm!"
Elizabeth, 28, advertising sales manager

"He was French (of course). He described my vagina and clitoris in French while we did it. I went wild."
Annie, 62, writer

" Just discovering every nook and cranny and finding that spot that makes my back arch in pleasure."
Murphy, 60, artist

He Knew How to Use Both His Tongue and His Fingers

Don't think that oral sex means you use only your tongue to give her pleasure. Creative lovers use every tool at their disposal. Many women love the feeling of penetration while they're getting oral sex, so while your tongue's performing its magic, bring your fingers off the bench. Here's how some men have successfully served their women a combo platter:

"He flicked my clitoris with his tongue, and then guided his tongue toward my vaginal opening, licking and probing, while using his finger to stimulate the clitoris. He alternated his tongue and finger. I believe he ended with his tongue on the clitoris. Heaven!"
Pearl, 22, chemist

"One finger pushing hard into my G-spot (harder than I'd ever think to ask for) while sucking on my clitoris (rather like a tongue-kiss) . . . YES!"
Ulla, 29, performer

"He licked my clitoris lightly while lightly fingering around the opening."
Zelda, 26, actress

"He massaged the spots on either side of my vagina with the balls of his thumbs while gently sucking on my clit with his lips."
Caroline, 29, teacher

"Long, slow, hard strokes of the tongue with tug on the clit at the end of each stroke, combined with two fingers inside."
Michelle, 36, marketing project manager

Perhaps because its taboo nature makes it all that much more arousing, some women were sent into ecstasy when their guy's fingers visited the back door:

"He put a finger in the anal area and one in the vagina while giving oral."
Nana, 37, marketing manager

"He applied steady side-to-side tongue on my clit, with a finger in my pussy that then snuck around to tease and penetrate my ass."
Beth, 43, designer

"He traced a figure eight with a finger inside, hitting my G- or A-spot ever so slightly."
Arianna, 33, household engineer

Note that you don't necessarily have to restrict your finger work to her genitals to drive her wild:

"My guy had a way of stroking my entire body at the same time, as well as humming."
Judy, 59, clinical researcher

"I love to have him gently play with my nipples while performing oral sex. I climax over and over with this multiple stimulation technique."
Casi, age and occupation withheld

But the pièce de résistance of multitasking advice comes from Annette, the 44-year-old manager: "French kiss all over like you would French kiss her mouth. Then while licking, kissing, sucking her clit, put your two middle fingers inside her, palm up with your index finger and pinky curled back. Move your fingers in and out, fast and slow. Curl your fingers up and while inside stroke the area right behind the clit. Keep licking, keep stroking. It takes practice and coordination, but trust me, it works. I've done it myself!"

He Showed Me He Loved It

Of course, it's not only great technique that produces memorable oral sex. Remember what we said at the beginning of the chapter: Showing her how much you love going down on her might be the biggest turn-on of all. If she doesn't have to worry about your pleasure, she can focus on her own. That's what worked for several of our survey respondents:

> "He did it so enthusiastically that he took all the self-consciousness out of it. He acted like he just loved it and wasn't affected by the conditions down there, so I was able to relax and enjoy."
> **Emily, 30, attorney**

> "My experience is pretty limited, but the best oral sex I've ever received was from someone who just made it very clear how much he enjoyed it and really took the time to prove it."
> **Jennifer, 34, nonprofit worker**

He Blindfolded Me

Sometimes what makes for great sex is the unexpected. Blindfolds can serve two delicious purposes during sex: to increase anticipation and to allow sensory deprivation, which isn't a kinky lab experiment but a technique for depriving your partner of the sense of sight so she can focus on sensations (in this case, great oral sex). We wouldn't suggest pulling out a blindfold the first time you're in bed with a woman, but in a relationship where partners trust each other, blindfolding can be a sexy part of your repertoire.

"My boyfriend blindfolded me, very slowly opened my legs, and took his time," says Inara, a 46-year-old writer. "Between the psychological factor of being vulnerable and not knowing what was coming next and his skill, it was amazing."

Many different household items can be pressed into blindfold service: a scarf, a tie, or an airline eye mask, for example. If your partner balks, back off.

And Then There's the Grab Bag of Oral Techniques

One of the many great things about humans is the variety of activities that turn us on. One person's aphrodisiac might be another person's sleep aid. So it pays to fill your sexual toolbox, especially when it comes to oral sex. Need ideas? We've heard of cunnilingus techniques that run the gamut from "stamina" and "the guy had a pointy nose" to "eating me out anally" (anal oral sex?) and "He didn't stop until I was done!" Here are some other sizzling recollections:

> "He did everything sensitively and with great authority."
> **Melanie, 28, grad student**

> "He ripped a hole in the crotch of my panty hose with his teeth in order to get there."
> **January, 47, paralegal**

> "He actually found it, responded to me, and didn't try to chomp it off when I got excited."
> **Alex, 35, college professor**

"When he knew when I was about to come he stopped, then started up again in a few minutes. He repeated that until he was ready to let me have a mind-blowing orgasm. . . ."

Heather 28, travel photographer

"Ignorance. He was 18, had never gone down on a woman before, and had no idea what he was doing. As a result, he had no preconceived ideas about what he *ought* to be doing. He tried a little bit of everything until he found what worked. Best oral sex ever."

Bryn, 41, secretary

Not everyone could recall a great oral technique. Some had forgotten the particulars—"I can't remember, it just worked!" says Alexis, a 27-year-old marketing manager—while others had simply not experienced anything worth writing home about. "I'm still waiting," says Abbey, a 30-year-old designer. "He hasn't mastered this one."

But in the end, know that for many women, what makes good oral sex isn't a specific move. "It's not necessarily just about the technique," says 30-year-old Brianna, a marketing specialist. "It's the person who's doing it, and the general situation you're in."

Her Geography of Desire

Don't focus your oral attention only between her legs. Many other parts of her body will respond to the touch of your mouth. Not surprisingly, her breasts and nipples are prime real estate. Nearly 82 percent of our survey respondents said they love it when their partner licks or sucks their nipples. Go slowly, though: Some women hate to have their nipples played with. Start out by kissing and fondling her breasts, moving slowly to the areola (the sensitive brown area surrounding the nipple), and then the nipple itself.

Another 56 percent named their inner thighs. Other favorite areas were the perineum, the area between her vagina and anus, and yes, even the anus. But certainly don't restrict yourself to those areas. Some women love to have their necks kissed, licked, and gently bitten, with the spot where the neck meets the collarbone and shoulders being singled out for particular attention. "For me, I love a good lick down on the area between my neck and shoulders," says Adrienne, a 33-year-old graduate student. "Give it to me hard and like you mean it." In fact, you'd do well to explore her entire body, including her mouth, ears, toes, abdomen, and even the spot behind her knees. "I like to feel my man's lips all over my body," says 36-year-old Michelle, a management consultant.

In what other areas other than your genitals do you enjoy oral action?

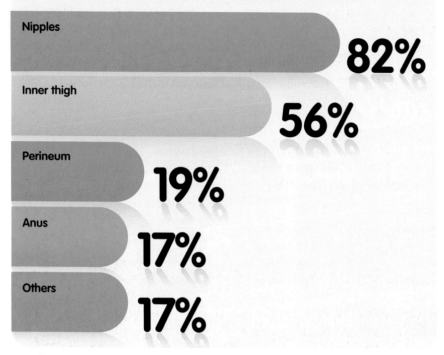

Nipples
82%

Inner thigh
56%

Perineum
19%

Anus
17%

Others
17%

Note: Respondents were allowed to select more than one answer to the question.

Which areas are off-limits for your mouth? For one, you might need to steer clear of her back door: Nearly 55 percent of our respondents want you to leave their anus alone, while almost 20 percent even want you to avoid their perineum. "Stay away!" says Marie, a 26-year-old teacher. Others, while not so definitive, still expressed some squeamishness, mostly around hygiene. "I still feel a little weird about it unless I'm totally fresh from the shower," says 46-year-old writer Inara. Other women mentioned toes and ears as body parts to avoid.

But for the rest—41 percent—there are no areas that are strictly off-limits. It's important to note that the more comfortable a woman is with you, the more likely she is to let you explore her body. For example, Roxie, the communications professional, said that while her bum wasn't off-limits, to her it's the "least interesting" for oral sex, and it "has to be the right person and time" before she'll let someone go there.

What Women Wish Men Knew about Fellatio

By now we hope you get it: Women like getting oral sex. But many men wonder whether their gals feel the same about fellatio. Well, rest assured that they feel good about it (as long as you return the favor—this is one case where it is quid pro quo). For some women, it is in fact their favorite thing to do. "This turns me on as much as him performing it on me!" exclaimed Pat, 56, project manager.

The following sections tell you what women want you to know.

Be Gentle, and Keep Your Hands Off Her Head!

Here's our number-one piece of advice about fellatio: *Hands off her head.* This is the one message that you should drill into your brain: Do *not*—under *any* circumstances—grab her head roughly, push it down on your penis, or hold it there. Yes, you've seen it in porn, but we have pages and pages of comments from women describing how much they hate this move. Here's a sampling:

> "I'm in control because I need to be able to breathe. Grabbing my head and keeping me down, or trying to dictate the speed of things, is a big NO-NO. By all means,

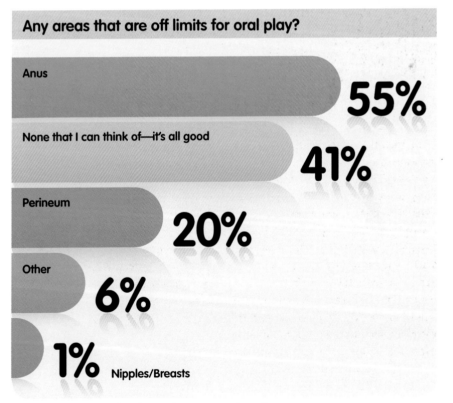

Any areas that are off limits for oral play?

Anus **55%**

None that I can think of—it's all good **41%**

Perineum **20%**

Other **6%**

1% Nipples/Breasts

Note: Respondents were allowed to select more than one answer to the question.

touch my head, touch my face, indicate you like what's going on, but don't you dare physically force my head to stay in a certain spot."
Adrienne, 33, graduate student

"What's with the head-grab-and-thrust thing some of you do? I am NOT a blow-up doll, moron."
Grape, 32, model/actress

"Stop pushing or holding a woman's head down there, either to get her to perform oral sex on you or to keep her down there!"
Helena, 39, professor

"Never, ever push my head down to initiate oral. I know where your penis is."
Michelle, 35, marketing project manager

"Don't force my head onto your penis really hard. I know how you can get into it—really exciting stuff down there—but if you put a little too much force on my head, then your penis jabs the back of my throat, and I don't like that kind of startling ram (although you may, in which case, get over it or find another woman)."
Carrie, 28, entrepreneur

"Head pushing would be a guaranteed good-bye."
Seraphin, 40, technology strategy

"Don't ever grab the back of a woman's head or hair and thrust into her mouth. Totally demeaning and unpleasant."
Scarlet, 34, chef

"Pushing my head down against my will is *not* the way to get me to perform it—it's insulting and a big turnoff."
Mae, 31, graduate student

"I don't want him to move my head with his hands. Better he holds my head gently and moves himself to the rhythm he wants."
Marisol, 66, writer

And while it's okay to show your pleasure by rocking your hips, be gentle. Do *not* jam, shove, or otherwise thrust your penis into her throat as though you're having intercourse with her mouth. ("I'm not Linda Lovelace" was a frequent comment.) Let her control the depth. Why? Well, have you ever heard of the gag reflex? It's something you want to avoid, because it's the quickest way to end a blow job—and not in the way you'd like:

"Don't have sex with our mouth. You'll choke us or make us throw up on you."
Jennifer, 30, banker

"Don't force it by thrusting into my mouth. I want to do it to you, not feel like my mouth is just another hole!"
Jane, 39, businessperson

"I need to be able to breathe! So don't think you need to choke me to prove how big you are!"
Pat, 56, project manager

"Keep your thrusting to a minimum, so we can have control over pace and depth. Nothing is more of a turnoff than almost gagging on some guy's cock."
Andrea, 40, administrative manager

"When I tell him to slow down, he should. I tend to gag easily, and sometimes they get into it so much that it's no longer fun for me."
Meagen, 37, psychotherapist

How do you feel about performing oral sex on a man?

I love it — **54%**

I'm neutral — **42%**

I'd prefer not to — **4%**

Note: *Percentages may not equal 100% due to rounding.*

"No matter how much I'm into it, it's gonna choke me if he gets too aggressive about his own pleasure, and neither of us is going to enjoy it."
Maureen, 45, archeologist

"If I want to take it in as far as it goes, I will. Don't push it."
Keite, 31, office manager

"Trying to keep my teeth out of the action requires a certain level of dexterity, and it's more difficult when a guy starts thrusting or moves my head."
Bryn, 41, secretary

We Do Like It—a Lot

Put any of your doubts aside. If your woman says she gets off on going down on you, don't second-guess her. She's telling the truth, so relax and enjoy. Twenty-seven-year-old Blair, a lawyer, says, "Sometimes guys get the impression most women don't like it and that it's just for them, but for many of us, we love it and enjoy it. And yes, some of us like to taste you, too; it doesn't gross us out." Adds Judy, 59, "Most of us really get into it. If we offer, let us!" Their enjoyment comes, in great part, from the bliss it gives you. "I love pleasuring my man, and I know men love this, so it makes me happy to do it," says Casi.

But, not surprisingly, a woman's excitement about this sex act has a lot to do with her feelings for the other person, the situation, and their mood. "I really enjoy doing it with someone I'm in love with," says Hailey.

What does this mean for you? Know that all women have different preferences. Suggests 44-year-old manager Annette: "All girls are different. Some like it; some don't. Some swallow; some don't. Take her lead. Don't push yourself on her. You'll be able to tell if she likes to do it or not. But pay attention and don't expect it. It's a gift." So let yourself go!

Give Us Feedback

Sex is a team activity. When it comes to fellatio, much of what turns a woman on is your reaction. So make sure you express yourself and tell her what you like—either by your ecstatic moans or specific verbal instruction. Give her feedback: Share what works and what doesn't, as well as what pressure and speed you need. And if you crave something in particular, clue her in. "Every man is different, so it's not a bad idea to let her know directly how to stimulate you," says Frankie, a 36-year-old swimming instructor. Adds Francesca, a 39-year-old education professional, "If there's something you like, tell me that before you complain that it's just not working for you."

Here's more advice:

> "Everyone loves a cheerleader. I'm paying attention to your breathing and your vocal cues to figure out what you like best, but you've gotta keep it coming. I LOVE pleasuring a man orally, especially when he makes me feel like I'm blowing his mind. The more you're into it, the more I'm into it."
> **Caroline, 29, teacher**

> "Tell me what to do! Is ball play okay or no? How sensitive/dull are certain parts? Is eye contact important? Do I go fast and hard right away? I enjoy doing it, and you should love that I enjoy it."
> **Elizabeth, 28, advertising sales manager**

> "His expressions and sounds are a huge turn-on and get me more into it."
> **Teresa, 33, marketer**

> "I like it more when I know you're into it, so tell me! Touch me while I'm doing it. You still need to be engaged."
> **Dawn, 29, public relations executive**

> "Please let me know if you like what I'm doing. If you lie there looking bored, it's no fun for either of us."
> **Inara, 46, writer**

> "Make noise. Don't leave me down there feeling disconnected and unsure if what I'm doing feels good."
> **Vanessa, 35, administrator**

> "I really do like doing it, but when I don't get any reaction from you, I get discouraged and will probably stop."
> **Roxanne, 45, writer**

> "Every man likes a different style. So when he says: 'Oh, this is so much better than four weeks ago,' it's because I figured out his preference."
> **Matilda, 32, pharmacist**

And give her some time to get to know your body and its responses. "If it's my first time with you, give me a couple of tries to get into a good rhythm with you," says Sara. "It changes for each guy."

Do a Little Manscaping

If you want to increase your chances of getting a blow job, you'd better be squeaky clean. Scrub all your nooks and crannies (and protuberances), because poor hygiene is at the top of the list of oral sex turnoffs. "You gotta be clean down there," 35-year-old Sheba, a lawyer, states. "If you haven't showered recently, don't let me go down there, because it's not fun!" Taylor, a 65-year-old comedy writer, puts it more bluntly: "A clean penis is a desirable penis."

So even if a woman doesn't ask you to do it, take a shower before you get busy. There's no need to dowse yourself in cologne (and please don't do that in lieu of taking a real shower). Says Inara, "The natural smell of a man can be a huge turn-on as long as it's a clean natural smell and not several days of 'I'm a manly man and do not need to bathe!' kind of natural smell."

It doesn't hurt to do some manscaping, either. "Please, please trim the surroundings if need be," says Shai, a 33-year-old marketer.

Remember That It Can Be Hard Work

Keep in mind that giving a blow job can be demanding physically, so have some consideration for the woman performing it. It's not easy having a penis in your mouth, after all. Despite our sincere interest in making you feel good, our mouths (especially our jaws) can ache after a while. "I enjoy it, but men don't realize how much effort a BJ takes," says Shelley, 38, an artist. "By the time you're done, your jaw hurts, you're tired, and they're not even that appreciative, though they are quite cajoling beforehand."

Above all, remember that there's a living, breathing woman down there. Stay connected with her. Look down and make eye contact with her every once in a while. "If I feel like I'm just a machine, like I'm masturbating you

with my mouth, I'd rather you just go ahead and do that yourself," says Emily, a 30-year-old attorney. "The guy should definitely get so turned on beforehand that he's about to go, so that the experience doesn't drag on."

So don't delay your release, and don't be upset if she wants to switch to a hand job or intercourse before you've had your orgasm. She may need to come up for air every once in a while.

Tell Us When You're Going to Come

Some women have no issue with you coming in their mouths. Others hate it. So be courteous: Give her a heads-up (no pun intended) when you're about to orgasm. "Although I enjoy oral sex and pushing a man beyond his limits, I'm not thrilled about his coming in my mouth," says 48-year-old Sylvia, a marketing rep. "I tend to take him to that point and deftly move my hand there."

In closing, remember, that even if she loves doing it, fellatio is her gift to you. "I only do it for a man I really love, so if I do it for you, be appreciative!" says Sally, a 29-year-old teacher. Adds Alison, a 36-year-old home-maker: "We will do it when we want to, not when you want us to." And if she doesn't want to do it on occasion? "Be respectful," says Yolanda, 35. "No means no."

Bottom line: Don't take the act, or the woman, for granted. Enjoy it, and let her know how much you appreciate her mouth work.

touch my head, touch my face, indicate you

Chapter 5

The Main Event

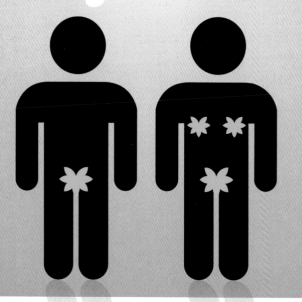

Doing it. Getting busy. Coitus. A bit of the old in and out. Boinking. The horizontal mambo/polka/tango/jogging/hula/hustle. You get the picture: We googled "euphemisms for sex" and came up with 1,710,000 results. (For the record, we particularly like the website Richard & Kitty's World of Sex Euphemisms.) Clearly, no other act between humans—heck, between any creature on earth—gets so much attention.

Whatever you call it, it means she's warmed up and ready to go, and so are you. We don't believe that intercourse should be the only focus of your time together, but let's face it, it's pretty darn important. We asked women to open up about the act. Is it good for them, and if not, how could it be better?

How often do women want sex, and are they getting enough? Where do they like to make love, and what's their favorite position? And then there's the question that's on every guy's mind when he gets naked with a woman: Am I big enough? Their answers will surprise you.

What Women Wish Men Knew about "The Act"

If your gal had to choose *one* thing that she wanted you to know about the sex act itself, what would it be? First, rest assured that women love intercourse as much as you do.

"Sometimes I have the feeling some men don't know that." Adds Susie, a 52-year-old marketing consultant, "It's my favorite—it's much better than anything else."

Other women noted its role in relationships. Rainna, a 56-year-old psychologist who has been married for more than 20 years, reminded men of its "importance to a vibrant marriage." In that same vein, remember, too, that sex is "a team sport," as education professional Francesca, 39, put it.

Now that we've got that out of the way, what were our respondents' top tips for ensuring that she *does* enjoy the act?

Focus on Her and Pay Attention

At the top of the list was a simple command: If you want to be a better lover, *pay attention*. Several women pointed out that believe it or not, sex isn't just about the man's penis and his orgasm. Gayle, a 33-year-old writer, pointed out that "sometimes it gets monotonous if my partner isn't trying to make sure I'm being pleased as well."

So follow her cues. Respond to her body. And not just because it's the sensitive thing to do. You'll increase your own pleasure tenfold. "Focusing on enjoying and pleasing your partner pays off big-time!" says 43-year-old Georgie, an editor. Adds Camilla, a 25-year-old advertising manager, "The more I enjoy it, the more you'll enjoy it too. I swear." Bottom line: Let your partner teach you what she wants. "Don't believe everything you see in the movies, and please don't learn about sex watching porn," says Jackie, a 50-year-old artist. "Get to know a real woman and find out slowly what she likes."

> ## "The more I enjoy it, the more you'll enjoy it too. I swear."
> **Camilla, 25, advertising manager**

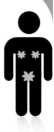

Take Your Time—But Also Know That Short Can Be Sweet!

Now that you're paying attention, what's the next thing women want you to know? Easy: *You need to slow down.* Take your time, guys. Enjoy the journey. Be patient. Yes, we know you're thrilled to find yourselves naked with a real live female, but remember that women aren't built the same as you are. Most of us take a little longer to get aroused—and to orgasm. "Let us have time to catch up to your excitement level," begs Judy, a 59-year-old clinical researcher.

If you don't focus some effort on getting her warmed up, you're almost ensuring a less-than-stellar experience. What's more, sex without lubrication can be uncomfortable, or even painful. "If it gets dry, there's no shame in using lubricant," counsels Pat, a 56-year-old project manager. But it's not only the physical discomfort that turns women off. "There's nothing more unsatisfying than jumping straight into intercourse," says Emily, a 30-year-old attorney. "It goes on and on and I either have to fantasize a scenario to finish or fake an orgasm." Like sports metaphors? Then heed the words of Mary, a 34-year-old consultant: "It's a marathon, not a sprint."

It's Not Just About the Sex

If all you're interested in is getting your rocks off, don't bother reading this. If, however, you're interested in really *good* sex and/or more than a one-night stand, pay attention. The act of sex itself, while definitely important, is not the end all, be all. Most women don't experience automatic arousal at the sight of your well-developed biceps or John Holmesian penis—they need more to get them turned on. Here's what our respondents had to say about the subject:

> "Sex is just part of the package. Pay attention to the whole person and you'll get lots more sex!"
> **Jackie, 50, artist**

> "Don't think about just this incident of sex, but how it will play out over the long run. Those who give will ultimately receive. Sex begins in a woman's heart and in her head. If you are not emotionally satisfying her, nothing you do in bed will matter."
> **Pat, 56, project manager**

> "If the woman feels comfortable with you emotionally, she will probably try anything you want."
> **Suzy, 32, business executive**

However—and this is a big one—"take your time" does *not* mean "pound on me for hours." Longer is not necessarily better. "It doesn't need to last forever" was a frequent comment. As Sophie, a 45-year-old designer, put it: "Duration isn't the way to give her an orgasm. If plugging away isn't working, try something else. Then get back to intercourse."

And we're not *just* talking about bringing her to orgasm—we're thinking of her general comfort, too. As we mentioned in the last tip, to really enjoy sex, a woman needs to get—and stay—sufficiently lubricated. "It can start to hurt after a while," says 45-year-old Maureen, an archeologist. "Be aware of her arousal level. It does fluctuate during the act itself." (And just to really confuse you, lubrication doesn't always mean desire, nor does the absence of lubrication equal lack of desire. It's just one of the crazy tricks our bodies play on us. That's why it's always good to—gasp!—communicate with your partner.)

But if you're both turned on and ready to go, there's also the joy of the quickie. "Sometimes 'wham, bam, thank you ma'am' is good!" exclaimed Marla, a 44-year-old singer. Elizabeth, a 36-year-old business owner, agrees: "Going for an hour isn't the goal. Sometimes short and sweet is awesome so we can bask in the post-sex glow."

Mix It Up!

How can you make sex more exciting for your gal? Mix up your moves every once in a while! In automotive terms, "There is more than one gear," says 48-year-old Ginger, a project manager. Again and again, the women in our survey said they want you to vary your rhythm, pressure, and speed. "Variations are good—like long slow strokes followed by deep penetration and back to long slow strokes," says January, a 47-year-old paralegal.

And your penis isn't the only instrument in your sexual toolbox (so to speak). Use your hands! Forty-year-old Andrea reminds you to "keep touching and showing interest in non-genital areas during sex or you'll lose my interest." Be willing to use multiple methods to ensure her pleasure, too: "Most women cannot orgasm just from intercourse, so try other things like vibrators and clitoral stimulation," advises Dawn, a 29-year-old public relations executive. After all, "you *can* have really good sex without the penis," says Annette, 42. "Lesbians do it all the time, and it's fantastic."

Variety isn't just the spice of life when it comes to techniques. Don't be afraid to try new and different positions, locations, and even the way you talk during the act. Your willingness to mix and match your sexual repertoire will pay off.

Gently Now

Another frequent comment we hear from gals is that (in general) you need to be gentle when touching and making love to a woman's body. "Harder does not necessarily equal better," said academic Alina, 25. Besides, "grinding, not pumping, creates orgasms during intercourse," says Taylor, a 35-year-old teacher. That's because grinding against her pelvis has a better chance of stimulating the clitoris, something that the old in-and-out doesn't always do. Remember, too, that her love button becomes ultrasensitive after she orgasms, so don't manhandle it after she comes, unless she asks you to.

And while there's certainly a time and place for crazed monkey sex (and you'll be able to tell from her body language whether that's what she wants), you miss out if that's all you do. "Take the time to enjoy it," says 22-year-old Pearl, a chemist. "The pleasure comes from the sensation, not the intense speed or force of the penis."

Communicate

How do you know whether she wants go-for-broke boinking or gentle lovemaking? Communicate, whether through words or body language. "Feedback, people!" says Lulu, a 35-year-old defense attorney. "You like it when we groan—we want to hear it from you, too!" Adds office manager Keite, 31: "Communication is key, even if it's nonverbal. Let me know if you like or don't like what we're doing." (In particular, let her know if you're approaching orgasm, so she can speed up or slow down appropriately.)

What's more, you might get some pleasant surprises. "Women might like something that you don't think they would like," says Heather, 37, a marine biologist. "So just ask if they'd like to try it. Hopefully, your partner has an open mind."

Being open about your needs—and finding out about hers—will benefit both of you, as Helena, a 39-year-old professor, points out. "I think that the best partners I've had recently have encouraged me to share what I know about my body and want to learn about me, my body, and how together we can connect best."

Put Your Heart—and Mind—Into It

You may have heard the old saying that 99 percent of sex happens between the ears. And for women (at least for our survey takers), this seems to be true. Time and time again, our respondents said that sex is an intimate, meaningful act for them and is "better when you have some kind of emotional connection," says 27-year-old Alexis, a marketing manager. In a committed relationship, sex is "mostly an emotional response, a gift," says Sylvia, a 48-year-old marketing rep.

"It's how I express my love for you, not just a thrill ride," says 33-year-old Arianna, a household engineer. Even the occasional quickie still has emotional aspects. "Yes, there are times when a woman just wants the sex," says 43-year-old Vicky, a professional water-skier, "but it'll be less than wanting the closeness and intimacy. Nine times out of ten it comes down to the caress and touch."

Some women, like 44-year-old Michelle, a stay-at-home mom, mentioned their need for an emotional connection—and your appreciation—outside the bedroom as well. "Romance makes it better," says Jenny, 28, a medical office manager.

Yet don't think all women need roses, soft music, and candlelight. "Women might be using you for sex just as much as you use them!" says Elizabeth, a 30-year-old advertising sales manager.

Orgasms Are Sometimes Just Icing on the Cake

Another thing women want you to know? She's not always going to have an orgasm, and that's perfectly okay with her. Don't take it personally, and don't pressure her. "Orgasms are not a life-or-death situation," says librarian Lula, 30. Adds Kate, a 34-year-old physician, "Women can thoroughly enjoy sex without actually having an orgasm." In fact, many women described orgasms as just one part of the whole experience, not the all-encompassing goal. Don't believe us? Hear it directly from our respondents:

> "Don't always expect me to have an orgasm. I like the act of sex itself."
> **Sally, 29, teacher**

> "Not all women will have an orgasm. Don't pressure her about it, but ask in a sweet way what she needs."
> **Nana, 37, marketing manager**

"Don't always expect me to have an orgasm. I like the act of sex itself."

Sally, 29, teacher

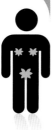

"We don't always have to orgasm to have a good time, but it sure doesn't hurt the cause."

Shannon, 40, travel writer

"Don't get too caught up in 'success' or 'failure.' Sometimes it's nice to just enjoy the ride without worrying about getting anywhere."

Marie, 29, scientist

Two other factors to keep in mind. First, her ability to reach orgasm may not have anything to do with you. Factors like medications, fatigue, and stress can affect her ability to achieve release. "I honestly do love sex, but I have to do a lot of fantasizing to get aroused," says Roxanne, a 45-year-old writer. "That's not a reflection of you but a reflection of my stress level and mental state, and the fact that I take antidepressants."

Second, remember that vaginal intercourse itself is usually not the best way to give a woman an orgasm, because most women need direct clitoral stimulation. You can increase the chances of that happening by changing your position to one where your pelvis hits her hot spot—or by simply using a vibrator or your fingers on her. As Beth, a 43-year-old designer, puts it, "Try to involve the clitoris in some way."

And finally, for some, good things come (literally) to those who wait. "I get turned on when my husband ejaculates," says Rose, a 30-year-old teacher. "Often if he can go for a little longer, I will have my most intense orgasms."

Does Size Matter?

Before we go any further, we feel we have to tackle the eternal question: Does size matter? We feel it's worth addressing in a chapter dedicated to intercourse because, at the risk of stating the obvious, the penis plays a big role in most definitions of The Act (those that involve a man, anyway). And we know that there's probably no question that causes more angst for you guys than whether your penis is big enough to give your partner pleasure. If this weren't the case, we'd be getting a lot less spam for penile enlargement pills in our email inboxes.

The thing is, you're probably not a good judge of your size. A lot of men underestimate the size of their penis because they're *looking down* (it's called "foreshortening"). So what do women *really* think about when it comes to penis size and intercourse? Does it matter?

Well, yes, said about 47 percent of our survey respondents, but—and here's the key part, so pay attention—*only* if their partner's unit is too big or too small (and even those are relative terms, considering that scientists can't agree on the "average" size of the male penis). For 38 percent, a too-small penis isn't as enjoyable during sex. For 9 percent, it's a too-large member. But what's important to note is that these women—along with most of the 25 percent who chose "other"—say that a love wand that's on either end of the size spectrum presents challenges during intercourse. "Too big can hurt and too small can be unsatisfying," says Shelley, a 38-year-old artist. It's not just the physical attribute itself that can be a problem.

In sum, "average" is just fine, thank you very much. "I've been with men with penises that are too small to feel, and men with penises that were too long and rammed up against my cervix and who had a difficult time being gentle enough for me," says Georgie, a 43-year-old editor. For some women, it all comes down to girth. "If the penis is literally like a pencil then it's difficult for me to figure out how to work with it," asserts Vicky, a 43-year-old professional water-skier. The other extreme poses a problem as well: "I used to go out with a guy who had a Coke can in his pants," says domestic executive Dawn, 42. "Holy crap, anything was painful!"

Basically, what it all comes down to is how well the two of you are matched physically. "I like the perfect fit," says artist Marla, 30. Adds 32-year-old model/actress Grape, 32, "I dated a guy for ten years faithfully, and we both got off so easily—he was medium-sized to small but hit everything right in me."

Women aren't comparing you against some standard of physical perfection either, so don't be self-conscious if your little man isn't perfectly straight when he's standing at attention. "A little bend in the dick is nice because hits the right spots," Marla says.

Remember, it's not the size of your member that counts. It's what you do with it that matters.

> **"Penis size only matters if all you are doing is intercourse."**
>
> **Rachel, 45, entrepreneur**

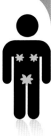

Does size matter?

YES:
If his penis is too SMALL, it's not as enjoyable — **38%**

NO:
It's what he does with it that matters — **28%**

Other — **25%**

YES:
If his penis is too BIG, it's not as enjoyable — **9%**

Note: Percentages may not equal 100% due to rounding.

Ginger, a 38-year-old project manager, summed it up: "I can come with or without a penis, but his control of the situation is critical. There is more than one way to please a lady." In other words, attitude is everything, as these women point out:

> "Men, gifted or otherwise, can learn to compensate for length, girth, etc., if they're willing to try."
> **JUDY, 59, CLINICAL RESEARCHER**

> "If it's too long, too short, or too narrow, then you just have to compensate with more clitoral stimulation."
> **DAISY, 40, STAY-AT-HOME MOM**

> "Penis size only matters if all you are doing is intercourse."
> **RACHEL, 45, ENTREPRENEUR**

Location, Location, Location

Where do women most like to hook up? For more than half of our respondents, the bedroom is where it's at, making it by far the most popular place to get up close and personal.

The Bedroom

This shouldn't come as any surprise, really. The bedroom is usually the most comfortable and private room in the house. "I can feel at ease and open there," says 41-year-old Bryn. Unless you have children, in which case you need to invest in a good lock, there's much less chance that someone's going to walk in on you when you're in your bedroom than if you're in, say, your backyard.

Some of the reasons women love their bedrooms: You can make as much noise as you want (usually) and the bed is the perfect surface for exploring a variety of positions. "There are good handholds!" says Kelly, a wildlife biologist. Postcoital cuddling is easy. You can store all of your nooky supplies—lube, condoms, toys—in your nightstand, within arm's reach. Best of all, if you fall asleep in your bedroom after sex, you're in the perfect spot to go at it again when you wake up.

So guys, if you want to really enhance your love life, invest some time and money in making your bedroom a place where your gal is actually going to want to spend some time. You don't have to bedeck the place with flowers and satin sheets (and we know how you feel about those stinky scented candles), but a dusty, underwear-strewn bedroom probably isn't going to get her in the mood. Keep it neat, comfortable, and simple.

The Great Outdoors

And if the bedroom isn't available, what then? Our survey respondents' second-favorite spot for romance was the great outdoors. "Good sex makes me feel alive and inspired; being out in nature makes me feel alive and inspired; together, that's a dangerously amazing combination," says administrative manager Andrea, 40.

There's something about being one with nature—whether it's a visit to the beach or a camping trip—that makes many gals want to be one with you. Karen, a 35-year-old student, describes what makes it so arousing: "At the beach, it's powerful to hear the waves crashing, or while camping, the wind blowing through the trees," she says. "There's just something inspiring about sharing the beautiful scenery with your partner, then wanting to add to that memory by sharing your bodies with each other in that setting."

Hotels

Coming in third place are hotels, whose major feature is—surprise!—a comfortable bed. "Hotel rooms *always* make me horny," says Caroline, a 29-year-old teacher. But a hotel room also allows women to escape everyday cares: Several gals mentioned not having to clean up afterward. Ellen, a 37-year-old Web development manager, expanded on the reasons: "A hotel has no kids, so there's no fear of being interrupted. It's private, but it's also a little bit public (people can hear through the walls), which is

What's your absolute favorite location for sex?

Bedroom — **54%**

Outdoors, nature setting — **12%**

Hotel — **9%**

Other — **6%**

Somewhere public where we can be discovered — **5%**

Living room — **4%**

Bathroom — **4%**

Jacuzzi or hot tub — **3%**

1% Swimming pool

1% Outdoors, at home

1% Kitchen

0% Someone else's house; office/at work; in the car; outdoors, urban setting; laundry; dining room

Note: Percentages may not equal 100% due to rounding.

kind of hot. I'm also usually on vacation when I'm in a hotel, so I'm relaxed." One of your coauthors began laughing when she read this, because at the time, she was on her way across the country to a wedding, which meant she would be spending three days in two hotel rooms with her husband and three-and-a-half-year-old son. "No kids"? Not always.

Other Places

A small percentage of women get turned on in a "public" place where there's a risk they might be discovered. One of these adrenaline junkies is 30-year-old Abbey, a designer: "My husband is less inclined to go for it in a public place, so I rarely get to take advantage of it," she says. "But the few times that we've done it have been so hot. I need something to make sex surprising again, and that's a great way to do it." (It's also a great way to get arrested, but that's part of the thrill, we suppose.)

Other places where women like to get it on include a chair, in front of the fireplace, and even at a sex party. Lula, a 30-year-old librarian, has more culinary inclinations: "Kitchen sex for us is usually totally spontaneous and quick, and I like the idea that he somehow winds up turned on watching me do dishes," she says. "I'm strange." Several frisky ladies said their favorite place for sex was "anywhere!" As Heather, a 25-year-old

executive assistant, puts it, sex is "the best when it's spontaneous and you just *have* to have sex then and there."

Some women noted that their preferences have changed over time. "I used to enjoy the outdoors and public areas, but less so now," says Sam, a 35-year-old lawyer. Pat, a 56-year-old project manager, says that her favorite place for sex "used to be the car, but at my age, comfort matters!"

Reality Locations versus Fantasy Locations

So where have women actually *had* sex? In our survey, at least, the most common spot was the bedroom, of course, followed by a hotel, the bathroom (including the tub and shower), the living room, a car, outdoors, someone else's house, and the kitchen. A little more than half of our respondents had enjoyed aquatic loving in a Jacuzzi, hot tub, or pool. And nearly half have done it someplace where they might have been discovered.

There were more exotic locations for love as well. Our survey respondents have had sex in a limo, a restaurant, a tree (a *tree*?), the garage, the student lounge, a library, an airplane (hello, Mile-High Club!), on a golf course, and even "at a porn shop in their movie-watching booth"!

In what locations have you actually had sex?

Location	Percentage
Bedroom	100%
Hotel	95%
Living room	94%
Bathroom	94%
In the car	83%
Outdoors, nature setting	76%
Someone else's house	63%
Kitchen	62%
Jacuzzi or hot tub	58%
Swimming pool	57%
Outdoors, at home	51%
Somewhere public we can be discovered	48%
Dining room	48%
Outdoors, urban setting	36%
Office/at work	30%
Laundry	24%
Other	10%

Note: Respondents were allowed to select more than one answer to the question.

Can We (Dirty) Talk?

We know that men like it when a woman expresses her pleasure during sex. It lets them know they're doing something right, and who doesn't like to get positive reinforcement? Certainly the women in our survey do—33 percent said they want encouragement when they're on the right track. Another 24 percent get turned on by moaning and other nonverbal demonstrations of lust. So don't be shy about moaning a nice "oh baby, yes, right there" if you like what she's doing. And compliments are always appreciated. "I find that the man complimenting my body makes me feel sexier," comments Shai, a 33-year-old marketer.

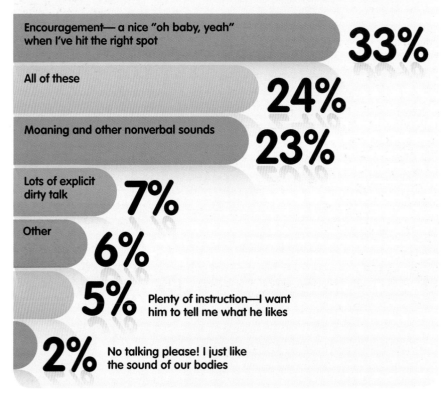

What kind of verbal action do you like during sex?

- Encouragement— a nice "oh baby, yeah" when I've hit the right spot **33%**
- All of these **24%**
- Moaning and other nonverbal sounds **23%**
- Lots of explicit dirty talk **7%**
- Other **6%**
- **5%** Plenty of instruction—I want him to tell me what he likes
- **2%** No talking please! I just like the sound of our bodies

Note: Percentages may not equal 100% due to rounding.

Despite what you might see in porn, explicit dirty talk isn't as popular—only about 5 percent of our respondents like that sort of verbal action. "I don't mind a little encouragement, but I don't like dirty talk unless I'm really into it . . . like when I'm buzzed!" says Marie, a 26-year-old teacher.

And if you need to give her pointers during the act, your best bet is to use a mix of gentle verbal pointers mixed with nonverbal cues—for 74 percent, this kind of instruction works best. Just don't turn into a drill sergeant. "A few verbal instructions are fine, but too many get annoying," says Heather, 25. On the other hand, some women do crave direct orders.

"I love it when my boyfriend takes charge sometimes and tells me what to do," says Inara, 46, a writer. "He gets this low, growly type of voice that totally turns me on."

What kind of instruction do you want him to give you during sex?

Combination of verbal and nonverbal cues — **74%**

Nonverbal cues (moans and pressure are good) — **13%**

Keep the instructions coming—I like to know what pleases him — **9%**

Other — **2%**

1% Stop talking—I know what I'm doing

Note: Percentages may not equal 100% due to rounding.

Favorite Positions

Time to assume the position! The question is . . . which one? Artists and pornographers have reveled in portraying human bodies coupling in all sorts of acrobatic contortions, but what works for the average person is quite different. We asked women to name their favorite position for sexual intercourse.

Interestingly, there was no clear winner—women were almost equally divided between missionary (face-to-face) and woman on top. For some, any position is a good position. Household engineer Arianna, 33, says she loves "all of the above and then some!" Administrative manager Andrea, 40, says, "I like so many positions, I can't really pick just one. I tend to orgasm more when I'm on top though, so that's always fun!"

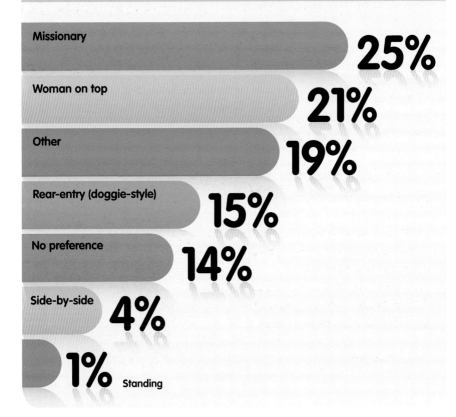

What's your favorite position for sexual intercourse?

Position	Percentage
Missionary	25%
Woman on top	21%
Other	19%
Rear-entry (doggie-style)	15%
No preference	14%
Side-by-side	4%
Standing	1%

Note: Percentages may not equal 100% due to rounding.

Missionary Position

You can't go wrong with the missionary position. Women love this old standby—face-to-face, with him on top—even more than being on top, which we thought would be the favorite because of the control it affords. About 25 percent of our survey respondents picked it as their favorite, citing the intimacy that this position affords—the eye-to-eye contact, the feel of skin against skin. "I like all positions, but I like the missionary position the best because it gives more scope for the man to kiss me, touch me, and make eye contact with me," says Allison. "I like to feel there's some emotion involved when I'm having sex." Others mentioned the sense of safety and nurturing they feel.

But several women named missionary as their favorite for more practical reasons—it's this position that has the most potential for getting them off due to the deeper penetration and better stimulation it allows. Some examples:

"My husband can take charge (I'm usually dominant in our day-to-day lifestyle), I get off more easily, and I can concentrate on the feelings rather than on my knees (me on top) or arms (doggy style) giving out. My husband can control his orgasm, meaning he has more staying power. The biggest reason is that his penis feels great and rubs my G-spot . . . just wow!"
Pearl, 22, chemist

"Missionary style is one of my favorite positions because with the right movements, a man can rub my clitoris with his pelvis while he's inside me. It's great for both parties when I can climax this way."
Adrienne, 33, graduate student

"Missionary position allows me to wrap my legs around his legs and pull his buttocks in for maximum pressure when I need it."
Sasha, 44, business executive

"I prefer missionary style because my partner can penetrate most deeply in that position."
Rose, 30, teacher

"I like missionary because it's a good angle for reaching my G-spot and because most partners I've had come too quickly if I'm on top."
Keite, 31, office manager

"Missionary style is my favorite because when he's on top, his body weight adds pressure to my pubic and stomach areas, which helps me to reach orgasm."
Vicky, 43, professional water-skier

Woman on Top

For similar reasons, many women like being on top during sex. (In Cynthia's book *What Men Really Want in Bed*, this position was actually the favorite of the men we surveyed. They liked the view.) For many women, being on top allows them to control the pace, the angle and depth of penetration, and the stimulation to their clitoris—making an orgasm almost a certainty. "Woman on top stimulates something that the other positions don't," says Sheba, a 35-year-old lawyer. "It's the only way that I can have an orgasm during intercourse." Here's a representative sample of comments we got:

> "I'm small and I can more comfortably receive and guide his penis in this position, which gives me a bit more control. And I've found it to be more pleasurable, i.e., the angles."
> **Embe, 52, bodyworker**

> "I can control the speed and point of contact. And I can slow him down or speed him up depending on where I am in the process."
> **Carrie, 28, entrepreneur**

> "I like being on top because it feels the most comfortable, I get to be in control, and men seem to love letting us do all the work."
> **Sara, 27, CPA**

> "I'm in control of the pace and the rhythm, and an orgasm is a 100 percent certainty for me."
> **Christina, 32, marketing manager**

Some women also like this position because it offers better access to her clitoris for both parties. "By sitting on him, I can masturbate or have him touch me at the same time," comments Stacey, a 33-year-old marketing professional. There's also the option of getting other erogenous zones involved: "If I'm on top, there's a chance for simultaneous clit stimulation and a finger in ass," says 43-year-old Beth, a designer.

Rear Entry

And, of course, there's the rear-entry or "doggie-style" position, which 15 percent of our survey respondents picked as their favorite. For them, this position has a variety of advantages: It feels the best, it allows deeper penetration, and it allows either party access to the clitoris. "It allows his hands to be free to continue roaming," says Sylvia, a 48-year-old marketing representative. "I like being on top for the same reason." Several women pointed out that rear entry also increases the chance of the man's penis hitting the G-spot. Some sample comments:

> "When I'm lying on my stomach, rear entry gives me the best orgasms."
> **Amy, 30, scientist**

"Rear entry excites me the most, due to the anticipation, and how the other person looks when you twist around." **Ursula, 39, astrologer**

> "I can hold the vibrator on my bits. They like that."
> **Dawn, 42, domestic executive**

> "It puts me more in charge of the movement without having to do all the work!"
> **Ulla, 29, performer**

> "There's something very animalistic about that position, and I love it when my boyfriend plays with me while he's fucking me."
> **Inara, 46, writer**

> "Doggy style definitely needs a better name, but it just feels the most like sex to me."
> **Maren, 34, physical therapist**

> "It feels good and looks hot."
> **Leilani, 31, pharmaceutical sales rep**

A few women mentioned exciting variations on the standard woman-on-hands-and-knees rear-entry position. Bryn, a 41-year-old secretary, describes her favorite position as the "mermaid": "rear entry, with the woman's legs together and the man straddling her legs. Putting a pillow under the woman's hips usually helps get the right angle." Stay-at-home mom Daisy, 40, likes a position that combines side by side and rear entry, defined as "woman on her back, man on his side, coming in from behind, kind of. Great access to all goodies."

It's a Toss-up

But for many of our survey takers, the position that ranks as their favorite all depends on their mood. For a romantic, intimate encounter, missionary or side-by-side position fits the bill. For more intense, spontaneous encounters, it's all about doggie-style, which women like Sunny, a 36-year-old project manager, describe as "nastier":

> "Missionary is the most intimate, and woman on top is great because he can have his hands on my ass and play with my breasts while I ride him, but a man almost always feels bigger to me when he enters me from behind. So when it's time to go all out and fuck, it's gotta be doggie-style."
> **Caroline, 29, teacher**

> "Missionary is the most intimate in my opinion, because you can look into each other's eyes and have your whole bodies pressed together, but doggie-style does more in terms of raw stimulation."
> **Mae, 31, graduate student**

> "I like doggie when I'm feeling naughty and lusty, and missionary when I'm feeling romantic."
> **Annette, 44, manager**

"If I'm in a mood where I want to climax, I like missionary, because for some reason my orgasms mostly only happen in this position. But if I'm not in the mood, I'd rather lie belly down, with the man entering me from behind. I find guys climax really easy in this position, so it ends quicker."
Shai, 33, marketer

"Preference varies by situation and person. For a hurried and surreptitious encounter, doggy; for a loving relationship, side-by-side."
Maureen, 45, archeologist

Some women's preferences vary with the time of day. "I like side-by-side in the morning, missionary in the afternoon, and for the evening session, a few ending with doggie," says Grape, a 32-year-old model and actress.

And for several other gals, it all depends on anatomy: "It depends on the guy, how he moves, and the size and state of his penis," says 40-year-old Seraphin, a technology strategist. But it's not just the man's equipment that affects their preferences: "My body has changed, so I'm figuring it out," says swim instructor Frankie, 40. "It used to be on top."

But no matter which position is your woman's favorite, remember that anything done to excess eventually loses its novelty. Several women said that when it comes to sexual positions, diversity is the key. "Variety is essential," says Sophie, a 45-year-old designer. "Anything becomes routine after a while." So mix it up. Be spontaneous. And read the next section for a few ideas.

What She'd Like to Try

So now that we know which positions women love, it's time to find out which ones they would like to try. How can you mix things up, and will she appreciate it if you try? Easily, and yes. We seem to have surveyed an experimental bunch. "I'd like you to show me a position I haven't tried," says Keite.

Others see an unexplored world ahead of them. "There are tons of positions I'd like to try," says Michelle, a 36-year-old management consultant. "I have bought a deck of cards with fifty-two positions. I plan to work through all of them."

Several women mentioned that they'd like to explore standing positions, up against a wall while "wearing a skirt" or "in a public place," or on top of an appliance (the washing machine rather than the stove, we hope). The element of passion and spontaneity seemed to attract these gals. Others mentioned less risqué but equally erotic situations. Thirty-year-old Lula, a librarian, says, "I'd love to be flexible and strong enough to do it standing in the shower, but I doubt that will ever happen." (Have faith, Lula!)

A number of women fantasize about doing it in a sex swing, and there were a few mentions of yoga moves and Tantric sex. "I'd like to attend some kind of sexual exploration workshop with a partner to learn about synchronizing your breath, Kama Sutra stuff," says Helena, a 39-year-old professor. "I'm pretty open to trying just about anything with someone I trust."

And then there was what we call the position sampler. Women mentioned wanting to have sex in a bathtub, or try "backwards" sex, anal sex, or threesomes (admittedly not a position, but certainly involving a variety of them). Nor can we leave out the more acrobatic and fanciful positions, many inspired by *Sex and the City*:

"I've never used ropes over the bed—aerial sex—and would like to try that."
Grape, 32, model and actress

"Zero G in outer space, no gravity."
Carrie, 40, scientist

"Reverse cowgirl . . . the porn stars make it look so easy!"
Ulla, 29, performer

"I saw it on the *Sex and the City* movie: The man is behind the woman and they are both upright and kneeling. His hands are caressing her breasts and labia."
Karen, 35, student

"On a washing machine. At full cycle. Probably one without shoes in it."
Carrie, 28, entrepreneur

"I saw one on *Sex and the City* with Samantha and Smith, where he basically sat on her torso and she had her feet in the air. I have neck issues, so I don't know if I can, but it looks fun."
Meagen, psychotherapist, 37

What's the Frequency?

Do you wish you were having more sex? You're not alone—chances are, your partner does, too. People usually think that they're having much less sex than the people around them, which we can assure you is not the case. One global sex study found that the average American had sex 138 times a year. (Only the French have more.) That comes out to about 2.65 times per week. We explain the 0.65 time as when the kids walked into the room or one partner fell asleep.

And yet, more than 73 percent of the women we surveyed said they wished they were getting busy more often. Their reasons ran the gamut. One pregnant woman who wanted more sex mentioned that her husband was nervous about having sex, a common but unfounded concern. (Guys, if it's a normal pregnancy, you won't hurt the baby.) Long-distance relationships left many women craving more nooky: "My boyfriend lives in Boston and I live in NYC, and we only see each other once or twice a month," says Michelle, 36, a management consultant. "It's not enough, but at least I have my toys."

Others mentioned age-related differences. "At a certain age, men seem to slow down," says project manager Pat, 56, who's married to a man nine years her senior. "Sadly, this is the same age women seem to want more!" Although there's truth to the fact that men's libidos do slow down with age as their testosterone levels decline, beware. One of your authors heard this excuse from her 38-year-old boyfriend. A month later, he dumped her because he'd met someone else.

And then there's the problem of waning desire during a relationship, after the initial attraction period wears off. Erika, a 50-year-old writer and teacher, says that although she loves her husband and wishes they were having more sex, "we've been married for decades—we're just not that into each other." Clearly, couples need to work on their sex life throughout their relationship.

In a comment on our times, stress was a frequently mentioned libido-killer. According to one study, partners of people who work more than forty-eight hours a week report major problems with their sex life. (The only good thing about recessions is that sales of condoms and sex aids seem to go up, according to Forbes magazine, because people go out less.) "Stress tends to cut back on the amount of sex we have, and I miss the frequency of it," says Inara, a 46-year-old writer. "That being said, what we DO have is always fantastic." It's not surprising that stress has this effect. When you're stressed, your body is in constant fight-or-flight syndrome, producing the hormone cortisol. Although this served our ancestors well—it's probably not a good idea to take a sex break while you're being chased by a predator—in the modern world, constant stress causes a variety of health issues, including lack of desire.

Our overscheduled lives don't help our sexual relationships, either. "I wish I was having more, but it's probably my own fault that I'm not," says Heather, a 29-year-old pastry chef. "I need to make more time for it." There's a good reason she's not, though: No doubt she's just exhausted. "I want more, but sometimes I'm so tired I turn him down," said Sheba, a 35-year-old, lawyer. Guys, know that your woman probably isn't happy with this state of affairs. Several women regretfully bemoaned their lack of desire. "I also wish I *wanted* to have sex more," says Alex, a 35-year-old professor.

On the other hand, there were those for whom no amount of sex would be enough, especially after going without. "Once you awaken the beast inside, I'm hungry for more," says Roxy, a 31-year-old administrator. "When it's dormant for a while, I don't crave it as much."

For some, it was a question of quality, not quantity. "I wish I were having more good sex and less mediocre sex," says Bryn.

Not surprisingly, many single women want more sex. "Lack of sex is the worst part of being single," says 32-year-old Christina, who works in marketing. This held true across all ages and situations. "My guy died a year ago, and oh, how I miss sex," says clinical researcher Judy, 59. And despite what popular culture might have us believe, most women aren't looking for random hookups. "I don't have sex unless I'm in a monogamous, committed relationship, so yeah, more would be nice," says Sara, a 27-year-old CPA. These women are independent and selective, not desperate. "I'm abstaining until I find the right man," says Karen, 35. "I'm not settling for less just to get serviced. I can do that on my own!"

Only *one* woman said that she wished she were having "less" sex. The rest, well, they're perfectly fine, thank you very much—often because they were in the throes of a new relationship. "Oh! That I could have met him sooner!" gushed Seraphin, a 40-year-old technology strategist. Others simply had found their sexual match: "At age 44, I finally found someone who wants to have sex as much as I do," says Annette.

How satisfied are you with how often you have sex?

I wish I was having more sex — **73%**

I'm perfectly satisfied — **26%**

1% **I wish I was having less sex**

Note: *Percentages may not equal 100% due to rounding.*

Who tends to want more sex more frequently: you or your partner?

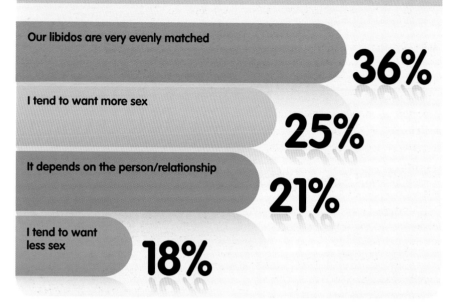

Our libidos are very evenly matched

36%

I tend to want more sex

25%

It depends on the person/relationship

21%

I tend to want less sex

18%

Note: Percentages may not equal 100% due to rounding.

Now that we've established that women love sex and generally want more than they're having, let's look at how that plays out in their relationships. Is the world filled with horny women and apathetic men? Not at all. Nearly 36 percent of our survey respondents felt that their libidos matched their partners', while about one-quarter claimed that they tended to want more. "I've never been with someone who wanted more sex than me," says Camilla, 25. "I think it's a common misconception that women want less sex. If it's good sex, girls want a lot of it, too!"

Unfortunately, some women find themselves feeling guilty about the mismatch in desire. "I feel bad if I'm always initiating," says Annette, 44. Others, like 45-year-old Roxanne, end up taking it personally. "I can't even say that my libido is that high," she says, "but I seem to want to have sex more than my husband, which has a negative effect on my confidence."

Some women find that their level of desire shifts based on a variety of factors: the situation, their partner, even the time of month. Again, modern life intrudes. "I used to want sex more," says Rachel, a 45-year-old entrepreneur. "But now I'm too busy."

Only about 17 percent of the women we surveyed admitted to wanting sex less than their partner did. Remember, though, that women can't go from zero to sixty in ten seconds. "Once I get going, I love it," says 26-year-old Marie. "Sometimes I need a little convincing." Important note: This is *not* to say that you should pressure or coerce your partner into having sex with you. It *is* a reminder of the importance of foreplay, paying attention to her feelings, and showing her how much you desire her.

For many women, sex is a reflection of the relationship. Says Allison: "Generally, I want it a lot, but if the relationship is going badly the sex life is usually going downhill, regardless of how attractive the other person is." (This reminds of us a picture we saw of a gorgeous man with six-pack abs. Below it was the caption: "Somewhere, somebody is sick of putting up with his shit." Remember this when you fantasize about being married to a supermodel.)

So what's a guy to do? Be honest about your desires—you may find that the two of you are more in sync than you realize. "I've had men reveal to me after the relationship ended that they had wanted more sex—but they didn't mention that when we were together!" complains Mae, a 31-year-old graduate student.

But don't push. If her libido seems to have flagged, try to find out what's bothering her. Is she stressed? Offer to put the kids to bed one night, and clean the kitchen. Never underestimate the value of "choreplay," which is one of the most powerful aphrodisiacs, according to women ranging from students to the wife of a high-powered executive.

> **"I think it's a common misconception that women want less sex. If it's good sex, girls want a lot of it, too!"**
>
> **Camilla, 25, advertising manager**

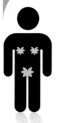

Crashing and Burning:
A How-To Guide

What's the best way to turn a woman off? If you want to ensure that she never does the deed with you again, try some of these moves.

Avoid Any Hint of an Emotional Connection

Sex is, at its most basic, about connection. So what's the surest way to cool a woman's passion for you? Pretend she's not there and don't look at her, as though you were imagining someone else. Don't pay attention to her cues. Act bored, like you just want to get it over with. More than anything else, women cited their biggest turnoff as being "someone who loses connection with me and doesn't notice that I'm out of the game," as Beth, 43, put it.

Women want enthusiastic, expressive, creative partners who care about how they're feeling. "I think it's supersexy when a man is keyed into what I want and need and is turned on by that," says Julie, a 43-year-old artist and writer. So at all costs, you want to avoid what Camilla, 25, described as "boring, fast, in-and-out sex . . . like they don't even need your help to get it done."

Have Sex Out of Obligation

The evil twin of emotional disconnection? "Rote lovemaking," says Karren, a 45-year-old attorney. Women can tell when you're having sex with them out of obligation. They hate "feeling like we're just doing it because we're supposed to have sex every so often, not because it's really desired," says Pat, 56, a project manager. So if you're not in the mood, be honest about it. If the word *should* crops up, it's a hint that you should *not*.

Make It All about You

Almost as bad as a lack of interest in her pleasure is focusing only on your own. "Self-absorption" and "selfishness" were cited by many of our survey respondents as being their biggest turnoffs in the sack. In a typical comment, Caroline, a 29-year-old teacher, describes that sort of guy who "makes absolutely no attempt (or a quick, limited, futile attempt) at making me come, and doesn't appear to care." Don't let this be you.

Pretend You're a Pile Driver

Passionate sex: awesome. Pounding away at her like you're a jackhammer: not so good. Women crave a gentle, lingering touch that starts with lots of foreplay and builds to a mind-blowing crescendo. As Inara, 46, a writer, puts it, she's not so psyched by "knowing that somewhere in the soundtrack of his mind, my partner is listening to 'Feels Like the First Time' while we're having sex and he just keeps pumping away forever with the same rhythm."

So vary your speed and rhythm. Swivel your hips. Change positions every once in a while. Remember that there are other motions than "in" and "out."

Take Too Little—or Too Much—Time

Although it's nice to delay your own pleasure so you can concentrate on hers, don't postpone the inevitable. Several women confessed to growing bored when their man took too long to climax—or refused to have an orgasm unless she did. "I don't need to go on forever," says Melanie, a 28-year-old graduate student.

However, don't attempt to set a speed record for fastest sexual experience, either. Women say they're frustrated by men who insist on "rushing it," or who finish too quickly. We know you're excited and all, but if you find yourself getting too close to orgasm, too fast, it's okay to slow down. Try pulling out and doing something else for a while. Then start up again. The good news is that if you delay your orgasm, the one you finally have will be that much better.

Talk Dirty to Her, But Not in a Good Way

Although some women like a little dirty talk in bed, others find what one woman described as "unwarranted dirty talk that sounds like it's from a porno" to be a complete buzz-kill. Marie, a 26-year-old teacher, says she's turned off by "really explicit accompanying dialogue. That's not my language, and it'll jolt me out of the mood quickly." Sure, it might be hot in the porn flick you watched last weekend, but this is real life. Take your cue from her. Start with a PG rating and then ramp up, seeing how she reacts.

Be Too Aggressive or Cause Her Pain

As one of our survey respondents said earlier, sex is a team sport—and you and your partner are on the same team. Unless you have specifically decided to explore BDSM (bondage and discipline, domination and submission, and sadomasochism) *together* and know what you're doing, treating her roughly is a no-no. Many women named "aggressiveness" as their biggest turnoff. Nana, a 37-year-old marketing manager, recalls an incident where her ex "thought because I wanted to try handcuffs that he should be forceful to the point of me becoming scared. He pushed me into positions roughly, and even though I told him my wrists hurt, he wouldn't take off the handcuffs. It seemed like a power play that I wasn't into."

In a similar vein, chances are that if it hurts, she's not enjoying it—so *stop*. Intercourse can be painful if she's not sufficiently lubricated or, more seriously, if she has a medical condition like vaginismus, or spasms in her vaginal muscles that can be caused if she's afraid that sex will hurt. Help her find out what's going on, and if the problem persists, insist that she see a doctor.

Have a Lazy Little Man

We were a little hesitant to mention this one, but some women mentioned a "soft penis" as a turnoff. Although this might seem cruel, we do have to admit that erectile dysfunction does tend to end the proceedings, which can be a letdown for all involved. However, there are things you can do. First, know that almost every man has trouble getting an erection at one time or another. You can avoid the problem by moderating your consumption of (or abstaining from) alcohol, nicotine, or cocaine. All of these can keep your member from standing at attention. Stress, anger, or unrealistic expectations can also work against you—yet another reason it's important to work on your communication with your partner.

Miscellaneous Turnoffs

Women also mentioned a few things that you'd have no control over—distractions like the phone ringing or crying babies; the wet spot—and some that you do, like inexperience (there are lots of books about sex out there, so read a few) or attempting anal sex when you haven't been granted permission. And then, of course, there was the grab bag of turnoffs: habits or problems that didn't fall into any specific overarching category, but that we had to list:

"Men who pretend they are IN LOVE with you to get you into bed. Just tell me you want to have sex!"
Francesca, 39, education professional

"Saying someone else's name."
Alexis, 27, marketing manager

"I dated someone who was way too melodramatic as he approached orgasm. I almost couldn't look at him."
Roxanne, 45, writer

"Once had a guy's belly flap (he had recently lost weight) smack me in the pubis during sex. SO not hot, just wanted it over!"
Scarlet, 34, chef

"Asking me to just tell him what to do to make me come, and not stopping despite me saying that I can't tell him that because I don't know. It's much more fun if a guy can just understand that I can enjoy sex even without orgasm."
Mae, 31, graduate student

"When you say 'hi' during sex. I finally said to this one guy, 'Who the fuck are you saying hi to?'"
Grape, 32 model/actress

"White socks that he doesn't take off."
Matilda, 32, pharmacist

"In missionary position, when I feel like I can't get any air. I'm mildly claustrophobic, so I sometimes get a little freaked out if he's 'in my face' for too long."
Bryn, 41, secretary

Parting Words

Please don't let this list of turnoffs discourage you. When we compared the comments we received to the attitudes Cynthia uncovered in *What Men Really Want in Bed*, we realized once again that men and women are more alike than different. We all want enthusiastic, passionate lovers who are thrilled to be naked in bed with us. We all want lovers who care as much about our pleasure as their own. (And we all want lovers who bathe regularly. But that's a given.)

Too often, we fall into the trap of believing that we should evaluate any sexual encounter by the quality of the orgasm. But sex is one activity where it really is about the journey, not the goal. In fact, we'd like to end this chapter with one of our favorite survey comments, which came from Annette, 44, a manager. "A big turnoff is assuming that intercourse is the ultimate act," she says. "If done well, everything *but* intercourse is the best part. 'The act' is just one of the many options. It shouldn't be the sole focus or goal."

Amen!

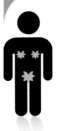

"It's much more fun if a guy can just understand that I can enjoy sex even without orgasm."

Mae, 31, graduate student

Chapter 6

All about Orgasms

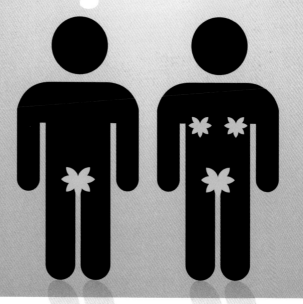

We asked several questions about orgasms in our survey, and originally, we were going to include the answers in chapter 5. But the more we thought about it, the more we thought that orgasms deserved their own chapter. After all, orgasms don't just happen during intercourse. They can happen during oral sex, from manual stimulation to genitals or other parts of the body (like nipples), with or without a partner, and even—for some very lucky women—from their thoughts alone. (True, but not common.) So what follows is a primer on how to give your gal a mind-blowing climax, as well as some tips on things that might get in the way of her ultimate pleasure.

In Search of the Big O

The female orgasm: easy or elusive? About 65 percent of our respondents said they have no trouble achieving orgasm; 34 percent admitted that they do. Medications and stress make the task more difficult: "The antidepressant I take makes it really hard for me to climax," says Roxanne, a 45-year-old writer. "And I'm under a lot of stress, which doesn't help, either."

It's worth mentioning once again that the majority of women need some sort of clitoral stimulation to climax. "I can orgasm during oral sex or manual stimulation, but never through penetration only," says Sara, a 27-year-old CPA. Despite what you might see in movies, orgasms during intercourse aren't the norm unless her love button gets some attention—which has a better likelihood of happening in positions like rear-entry or woman-on-top. "Vaginal orgasm is difficult, but possible," says management consultant Michelle, 36. "My current partner is aware of this and we are enjoying figuring out what it takes."But "yes" and "no" don't describe the picture quite accurately. We realized that we should have offered "sometimes" as an answer, because many women have trouble reaching orgasm occasionally, especially if they're stressed, lose focus, or aren't totally comfortable with their partner. "It depends on how much the man knows and his attitude about it," says song artist Heather, 31. "If he's good at pleasing me and encourages me, I don't have a problem. If he is impatient with me, I will not orgasm."

The message, guys: Pressuring your partner to have an orgasm—or to have an orgasm faster—isn't going to work in anyone's favor.

Do you have trouble reaching orgasm?

NO
66%

YES
34%

Note: Percentages may not equal 100% due to rounding.

Some women have no trouble having an orgasm through solo masturbation, particularly if they use a vibrator, but their climaxes take longer or are harder to achieve with a partner. "For me, orgasm rests in large part on the fantasy narrative inside my head," says Mae, a 31-year-old graduate student. "When I'm with a partner, I'm focused on him and not on fantasies so much. I still enjoy sex even without orgasm, though."

And even if a woman doesn't have problems climaxing, it may take her longer than you think. So be patient and don't rush her. "It takes a long time for me, but I'm fortunate to have someone who pays attention to what I want, asks questions, and experiments with various techniques and has now mastered what I like," says 44-year-old manager Annette. "I truly appreciate the effort of discovering what works for me."

Give Her Time to Unwind

Although there are some people who can switch gears from a stressful workday to sexual dynamo within seconds of walking in the front door, most women (in fact, most modern humans) need some time to transition between the two. If your partner just got home from a long and frustrating day at the office, give her a chance to unwind before trying to get her into bed. Better yet, offer a glass of wine and a sensual backrub to bridge the two moods. You'll both be glad you did!

> "Having some time to relax and rest before sex is very helpful. I can't go from stressful day straight to turned on."
> **Carrie, 40, scientist**

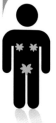

"For what it's worth,
I don't fake orgasms."

Troy, 29, lawyer

Do you let him know if you're having trouble reaching orgasm?

YES, so he'll try something else to make me come — **61%**

NO, I'll take care of it later — **39%**

Note: Percentages may not equal 100% due to rounding.

The problem is, although the majority of women will tell you if it's not going to happen for them, many women won't. About 40 percent of the women in our survey said that they keep quiet and take care of their needs later. (And yet, in Cynthia's book *What Men Really Want in Bed*, almost *all* of the men surveyed said they want to know so they can try something else.) So why don't women speak up? Several women mentioned that they don't want to hurt their partner's feelings or "kill the mood." In a typical response, 29-year-old Marie, a scientist, says, "If I tell him I'm not getting there, it'll ruin his mood, too—I want at least one of us to be happy!"

For others, it depends on the situation and the guy. Women who are comfortable with their partners tend to say something "so that he'll stop trying and we can get on with things," as writer Roxanne, 45, puts it. But if a woman senses it might harm your ego, she might keep quiet. "I always hope he'll manage it before it becomes really apparent, but usually that doesn't happen, so I always have to say that I'm a hard woman to please," says Allison. "It really has had negative impacts on a lot of my previous relationships when the guy gets insecure about it."

Other women don't say anything because, well, they assume you're aware of the situation. Says physical therapist Maren, 32: "He knows. They always know. Sometimes we talk about it, so he knows we don't have to try anything and everything to get there." Which brings us to an important point: Many women said they don't always need an orgasm to enjoy sex, so you shouldn't feel like you've failed if your woman doesn't climax once in a while. That doesn't mean you get to be rude and never take her desires into account. "But I hate when he thinks just because he's done, I'm done," says entrepreneur Carrie, 28. "If I roll over in exhaustion, I'm done. If I'm still up in your grill, I'm not done."

Surefire Orgasm Techniques

So if you want to make sure your gal has a good time, what are your best bets? First of all, learn where her clitoris is—and what she likes. More than 80 percent of our survey respondents said that clitoral stimulation (see chapters 3 and 4) is the best way to send her over the moon. Foreplay (lots of it—see chapter 2), oral sex, vibrators, and intercourse itself are also winners.

At the bottom of the list? Bondage, anal intercourse, role-playing, public sex, domination, and pain (although these did work for some women). All of these ranked after George Clooney as orgasm guarantees (and if you're wondering, George sends about 11 percent of our survey takers into paroxysms of ecstasy).

> "If I tell him I'm not getting there, it'll ruin his mood, too—I want at least one of us to be happy!"
>
> Marie, 29, scientist

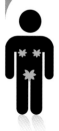

What are some surefire techniques that bring you to orgasm?

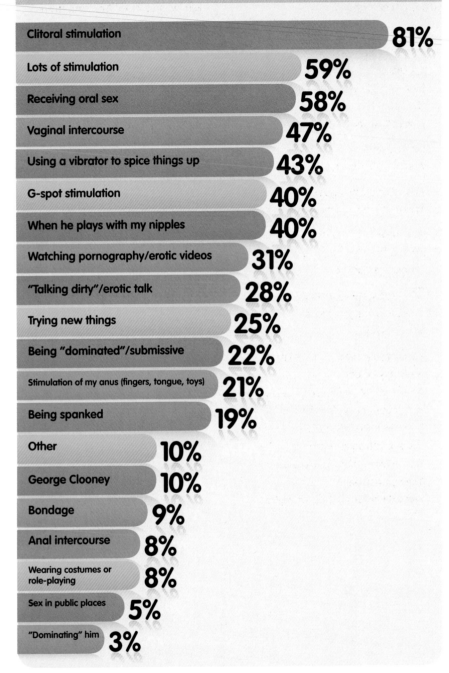

- Clitoral stimulation — **81%**
- Lots of stimulation — **59%**
- Receiving oral sex — **58%**
- Vaginal intercourse — **47%**
- Using a vibrator to spice things up — **43%**
- G-spot stimulation — **40%**
- When he plays with my nipples — **40%**
- Watching pornography/erotic videos — **31%**
- "Talking dirty"/erotic talk — **28%**
- Trying new things — **25%**
- Being "dominated"/submissive — **22%**
- Stimulation of my anus (fingers, tongue, toys) — **21%**
- Being spanked — **19%**
- Other — **10%**
- George Clooney — **10%**
- Bondage — **9%**
- Anal intercourse — **8%**
- Wearing costumes or role-playing — **8%**
- Sex in public places — **5%**
- "Dominating" him — **3%**

Note: Respondents were allowed to select more than one answer to the question.

Other techniques mentioned by our survey takers:

"I definitely have a thing for being 'taken' as long as there's no real pain involved. I love having my wrists pinned down to the bed very tightly. It's guaranteed to ramp things up."
Inara, 46, writer

"Lesbian porn."
Annette, 44, manager

"Masturbation during sex."
Frankie, 36, swim instructor

"Reading erotica, especially if it involves threesomes (two men, one woman)."
Roxanne, 45, writer

"Nothing's surefire, but erotic talk/books/movies go a long way."
Sam, 35, lawyer

"Watching him having sex with me, especially looking into his eyes. Also, long periods of not seeing each other (okay, two or three days, but whatever—time is relative). The best is nipple play, then oral sex with orgasm, then vaginal sex with orgasm. Then a drink of water. Then go at it again."
Seraphin, 40, technology strategist

"Deep penetration and ejaculation (without a condom). The warmth and movement of his penis during ejaculation stimulates whatever gives me the orgasm."
Shai, 33, marketer

"It's more about keeping focused on what's happening, rather than what is being done to me specifically."
Rachel, 45, entrepreneur

"I stimulate myself while giving oral sex."
Kara, 49, hairdresser

Clearly, the paths to orgasm are as varied as the women who have them. The only way you'll know what works for your woman is through trial and error—and actually talking to her to find out what she likes.

Faking It

So given that most women will, on occasion, have trouble achieving orgasm—and that they might not tell you—what, then, *do* they do? Unfortunately, nearly 75 percent of the women we surveyed admitted to having faked an orgasm. Their reasons varied: They were tired or drunk and knew they weren't going to climax, or they wanted to spare the guy's feelings. Twenty-five percent said they simply wanted to end sex. And 42 percent said that they've faked an orgasm for all of these reasons, at one point or another.

Some women end up faking it because they feel pressure to orgasm. "Men feel it's them if you don't have an orgasm," says Nana, a 37-year-old marketing manager. "The more they ask if I've had an orgasm, the more likely I am to fake it because I can tell they will feel let down. If it's a long-term relationship or has the potential to become one, I'll be honest and never fake it. But I have faked it during one-night stands."

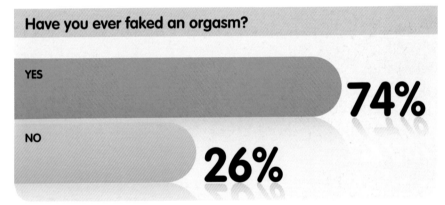

Have you ever faked an orgasm?

YES **74%**

NO **26%**

Note: Percentages may not equal 100% due to rounding.

If you faked an orgasm, what was the main reason?

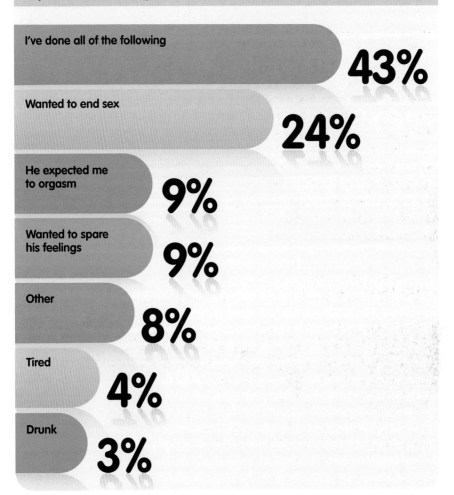

I've done all of the following **43%**

Wanted to end sex **24%**

He expected me to orgasm **9%**

Wanted to spare his feelings **9%**

Other **8%**

Tired **4%**

Drunk **3%**

Note: Percentages may not equal 100% due to rounding.

Others feel that their partner just isn't willing to go the distance with them.

"Getting me to orgasm takes some time," says Vicky, 43, "and unless they're willing to invest and make it happen, then most of the time, I put my needs aside. I've been with very few men who really want to understand and take the time to get me there."

It's a shame that so many women are willing to "put their needs aside"—especially because the majority of men don't want their partners to fake it, as Cynthia found in *What Men Really Want in Bed*. And many women agree that it's better to be upfront about your pleasure; to them, faking an orgasm sends the wrong message. "Why would anyone ever want to fake an orgasm?" asks Seraphin, 40. "He'll think he did fine and dandy rather than try to do better. Bad! Bad! Bad!"

We asked women how they'd feel if the shoe were on the other foot, so to speak, and their partner faked an orgasm. Half said that they'd be disappointed, but another 32 percent were surprised that it was even possible. Men fake orgasms? Well, yes, they do: More than *half* of the men who took Cynthia's survey for *What Men Really Want in Bed* admitted that they had—for the same reasons that women do. (And in case you're wondering, it seems that thanks to condoms and a little quick maneuvering, men *can* hide the fact that they didn't climax.)

> **"Why would anyone want to fake an orgasm? He'll think he did fine and dandy rather than try to do better."**
>
> **Seraphin, 40, technology strategist**

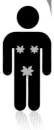

How would you feel if your partner faked an orgasm?

I'd be disappointed—he should let me know so we can stop or try something else — **49%**

Men can fake orgasms? — **33%**

It wouldn't bother me — **18%**

Note: Percentages may not equal 100% due to rounding.

What it seems to come down to is this: If you don't want your gal to fake her orgasms, spend a little time getting to know how her body works and what it likes. Become familiar with what she looks and sounds like when she does climax: Her breathing will speed up and become shallower, her nipples may harden, her muscles will tense. And when release comes, the muscles of her vagina will contract rhythmically, which you'll probably feel if you're inside her.

But even if you know the signs, don't make her orgasm a measure of your skill as a lover, the basis for your self-esteem, or the criteria by which you evaluate your sex life. Sometimes she'll climax; sometimes she won't, possibly for reasons totally out of your control. Whatever you do, don't pressure her or make her feel guilty if she doesn't climax. We know of one man who told his lover that she was "uptight" when she had trouble, which, we probably don't need to tell you, was not the way to send her over the moon.

The Truth about Multiple Orgasms

On a happier note, let's talk now about the opposite of a nonexistent orgasm: multiple orgasms! Researchers usually define this wonderful phenomenon as having two or more orgasms separated by only a few seconds, without your arousal level fading. "Some women (me) *do* have multiple orgasms from intercourse," says Erika, a 50-year-old teacher. "I'm not weird, and I'm not faking."

In our survey, 78 percent of women said they'd experienced multiple orgasms; 15 percent hadn't; and about 7 percent weren't sure. Why are multiple orgasms easier for women than for men? Blood flow. During a man's orgasm, blood quickly flows out, which is why men need a "refractory period" of rest before they can get hard again.

In contrast, blood flows in and out of a woman's genitals quite easily. After an orgasm, they stay engorged. So if you keep pleasuring your woman after her first orgasm, she may be able to come again. Try varying the type of stimulation you're giving her: Pull out of her and use just your fingers or tongue, or, if you've been making love missionary style, ask her to hop on top of you. Just know that her clitoris may be too sensitive for direct stimulation, so focus your attention on the surrounding area. She may feel at first that it's too much, but if you keep going (with her permission), you may both be amply rewarded.

But if it doesn't happen, it doesn't happen. Don't lose sight of the fact that sex isn't about achieving a goal. It's about giving and receiving pleasure.

Have you ever experienced multiple orgasms?

YES 78%

NO 15%

Not sure 7%

Note: Percentages may not equal 100% due to rounding.

"Some women (me) do have multiple orgasms from intercourse. I'm not weird, and I'm not faking."

Erika, a 50-year-old teacher

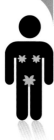

Chapter 7

The Afterglow

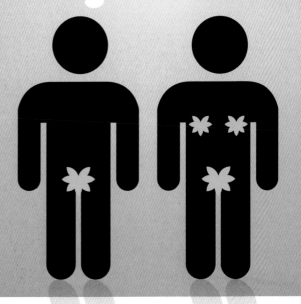

We've discussed seduction and the do's and don'ts that lead up to sex, and we've discussed the main event itself. Now it's time to tackle what happens *after* the deed is done. Our survey results will tell you what women are looking after sex: whether cuddling is important, how soon is too soon to roll over and go to sleep, and what kinds of inappropriate behavior will send them running for the door (or kicking you out their door).

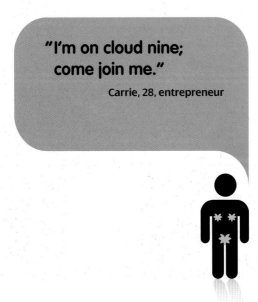

"I'm on cloud nine; come join me."

Carrie, 28, entrepreneur

What Women Wish Men Knew about the Afterglow

To cuddle or not to cuddle? That is the question. Whether 'tis better to suffer the snores and attention deficits in the postcoital afterglow or to go take a shower.... Well, you get the idea. We've all heard the common complaint about men rolling over and going to sleep after they pull out, or even worse, getting up and leaving (or expecting the woman to vamoose) when the deed is done. So we asked our survey respondents if after-sex cuddling was important to them. Here's what they said.

Take Some Time for a Little After-Sex Cuddling

The majority of our respondents—although at 43 percent, it's a slim majority—consider postcoital cuddling necessary for a positive sexual experience. We're not talking a full-on body massage or an analysis of the relationship here, guys. It can be as simple as pulling her against you to spoon and kissing the back of her neck, or brushing the hair off her forehead and telling her she's beautiful. A little goes a long way, as long as it's sincere. For some women, such as Sara, a 27-year-old CPA, it's mandatory. "Cuddling is required," states Sara, "as is not playing dumb about what we just did." Adrienne, a 33-year-old

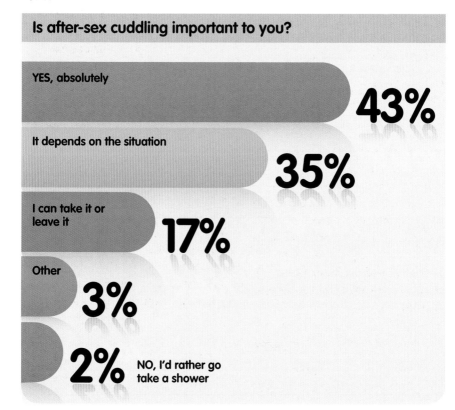

Is after-sex cuddling important to you?

YES, absolutely — **43%**

It depends on the situation — **35%**

I can take it or leave it — **17%**

Other — **3%**

2% NO, I'd rather go take a shower

Note: *Percentages may not equal 100% due to rounding.*

graduate student, says, "Let me bask in the glow and be there with me." Depriving these gals of after-sex cuddles is like taking a chocoholic out to dinner and telling her, sorry, she can't have the triple chocolate mousse for dessert because you're either too busy or just aren't in the mood for it. Makes for a lousy ending to an otherwise nice dinner.

Keep in mind women aren't necessarily asking for hours of extended cuddling, which is probably why 35 percent of the women in our survey said it all depends on the situation. Caroline, a 29-year-old teacher, explains. "I'm fully aware that men want to fall asleep after sex," she says. "All I'm asking for is a couple of minutes and a little bit of tenderness, and I'll leave you alone the rest of the night." Shannon, a 40-year-old travel writer agrees: "I'd like to be appreciated, but we don't need a lot of cuddling."

And sometimes it really is the thought that counts. Women want to know that you enjoyed what just happened. They don't expect a monologue; a "Wow, that was amazing!" will take care of it. Twenty-five-year-old Camilla, an advertising manager, explains, "I just want to feel loved and appreciated at that point. No need to talk or kiss or hug forever, just make sure I feel appreciated." Or, as 29-year-old performer Ulla puts it, "It's very rare that a girl is feeling as wonky and out-of-it postorgasm as you are. We almost always at least want the *offer* of a cuddle."

By the way, nonverbal expressions of satisfaction work just fine, thank you very much. Mallory, a 28-year-old mother, is fine with "at least a kiss or two. Some nice light finger tracing on the skin for a minute feels good, too."

That being said, there are always the exceptions, such as Karren, a 45-year-old attorney. "Not all women want to cuddle and talk after sex," says Karren. "Sometimes, I just want to wash off and relax with you beside me."

Talk to Her

Although not every woman wants extended conversation or even expects anything coherent to come out of a man's mouth after he's had an orgasm, there are some who do want more than snores or "thanks a lot, I'll call you" when all is said and done. As Leilani, a 31-year-old pharmaceutical sales rep, explains, "I love talking afterward."

Basically, women like to know—briefly—that you've had a good time, and to feel good about it themselves. Jackie, a 50-year-old artist, tells us, "It's a happy time. Enjoy it. Don't talk about anything serious, and compliment me on anything good I did during sex." Again, even just a simple "wow" will do. "I like to have a little cuddling and a little praise," says Jennifer, a 34-year-old nonprofit worker. Roxie, a 35-year-old communications professional, agrees: "It's a good thing to call it out—mention how much you enjoyed it and what you liked."

What women *don't* like? Feeling like they've been used. Fifty-six-year-old project manager Pat exclaims, "TALK TO ME! Whether it was good or not so great, treat me like a person rather than a blow-up doll!" Sasha, a 44-year-old business executive, adds that guys "need to remember you're still there and want to be spoken to and caressed."

Beth, a 43-year-old designer, has a gentler take on the topic of postcoital conversation. "It's a good time to enjoy each other as you both fall asleep. Talk, gently caress each other. Stay in the moment for a while."

Even If You Don't Talk, Try to Connect

Conversation, while important to a lot of women, isn't always the point. Indeed, for 25-year-old academic Alina, talking definitely is *not* the priority. "If it was good," says Alina,

"I'm still coming down from a high, so a little bit of quiet and light touching is better than engaging in full-on conversation about how good it was."

Sometimes it's just about feeling connected to your partner even after the last shudder of orgasm has passed. "We want to be held," says 27-year-old lawyer Blair. "And feel cared for and have that nice bonding time together." Adds Alison, a 36-year-old homemaker, "We feel really connected to you at that time, so don't belittle or break that connection too quickly."

Want a scientific explanation? We're glad to provide one, complete with a footnote, 'cuz it makes us sound so intellectual and all. Remember that her levels of oxytocin—also known as the "cuddle chemical" because of

> ## "We want to be held and feel cared for and have that nice bonding time together."
>
> **Blair, 27, lawyer**

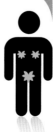

its role in promoting bonding—increase after orgasm, infusing her with feelings of well-being and making her feel closer to you. (At least that's the way it works for prairie voles, better known as field mice. One research study showed that oxytocin released into the brain of the female prairie vole during sex activity "is important for forming a monogamous pair bond with her sexual partner.") That's why your partner is in a state of "euphoria," as 35-year-old student Karen describes it. "I feel a strong emotional connection," she says. For Susette, a 70-year-old writer, the time after sex is a "time for closeness." Sunny, a 36-year-old project manager, puts it more bluntly, issuing this warning: "This is when I get the most clingy!" (At least she's honest.)

Connecting doesn't always mean talking. Roxanne, a 45-year-old writer, simply wants "silence and stroking" when the lovemaking is over.

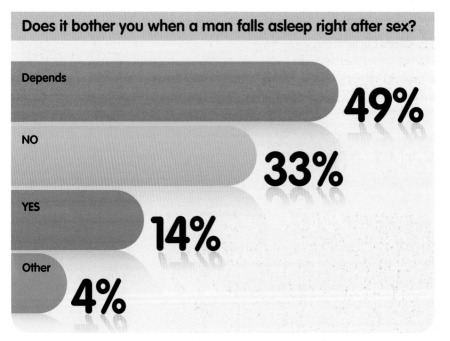

Does it bother you when a man falls asleep right after sex?

Depends **49%**

NO **33%**

YES **14%**

Other **4%**

Note: Percentages may not equal 100% due to rounding.

Recognize That We Get Sleepy, Too!

Most women know that men can't help the fact that they get really, really sleepy after sex. And for the most part, they don't mind, even if, like Leilani, they are "wide awake afterward," or "feel energized," like 49-year-old restaurant owner Monica. And it doesn't bother Mae, a 31-year-old graduate student, "whether or not I am ready to snooze myself." It all depends on the situation, according to about half of our respondents.

One reason we don't mind? Well, guys, unless we're like Leilani or Monica, men aren't the only ones who get groggy after sex. Nearly 33 percent of our survey respondents say they're ready to snooze themselves. Julie, a 43-year-old artist and writer, freely admits, "I like to go right to sleep, too!" And for Francesca, a 39-year-old education professional, the fact that her man conks out after sex is totally not an issue because "I usually fall asleep, so I can't complain."

That's why you shouldn't feel badly if you can't stay awake for hours (or even minutes) afterward. Says Heather, a 25-year-old executive assistant, "We *do* understand if you don't really want to cuddle all night long!" Just remember that a little cuddling goes a long way. Sally, a 29-year-old teacher, simply wants her man to "cuddle with me for a few minutes, say something nice to me, and be there with me. Then let's go to sleep!" Roxanne is even more low-maintenance: "I really don't need to talk after sex, especially if it's late at night. I'm tired, too!" Oh, and you might try and work on that annoying breathing thing. After sex, Amy, a 30-year-old scientist, says, "I like to roll over and go to sleep and not be breathed on."

> ## "We *do* understand if you don't really want to cuddle all night long!"
>
> **Heather, 25, executive assistant**

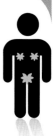

Unfortunately, whether your gal is down for the count or channeling the Energizer bunny seems to depend on the luck of the draw. Lula, a 30-year-old librarian, says, "I'm either going to fall asleep, or if it's morning sex, be very, very hyper. Deal with it." And Matilda, a 32-year-old pharmacist, says, "I'm actually usually very energized and want to do something like cleaning, etc. On the other hand, I am sometimes very tired and sleep, and in other situations I like to cuddle. It really depends." You'll either get a good night's sleep or a really clean house.

Relax and Enjoy the Moment

Sometimes it's not just about the particulars of what you do after sex, but also about what you don't do: Look at your watch, jump out of bed, run off to your next appointment, or commit other postcoital crimes. "Snuggling and chatting is nice, or a shower," says 35-year-old lawyer Sam. "Even sleeping is okay, but running off would be terrible." Rose, a 30-year-old teacher, agrees, saying, "Enjoy the glow. If possible, don't rush off."

The release of tension engendered by good sex is something to be savored together, at least according to Ginger, the 38-year-old project manager. For her, the time after sex is for "enjoying the release and not rushing off to do something else. I want to hear our breathing return to its normal rate." Like men, some women are blissed out after a good session of lovemaking and want a chance to bask in it. As Arianna, a 25-year-old household engineer, puts it, "If it was good, I am in a state of euphoria and don't want to move, but just relish the moment." What's the best part of sex for Sylvia, a 48-year-old marketing rep? "It's that closeness that comes afterward, the little touches, smiles, teasing," she says about her current relationship.

For many women, sex doesn't end with the orgasm. "Just like with your workouts, you need a cool-down period," says marketing project manager Michelle, 38. And Marla, a 30-year-old artist, has this to say about the postcoital afterglow: "Let's enjoy the rest of the day and bask in the beauty of love."

Don't Be Offended If She Heads for the Bathroom

Sometimes it's the man who wants to cuddle and bask in the languorous afterglow of his orgasm, and he doesn't understand why his partner insists on hopping right out of bed and hightailing it to the bathroom. Aside from the fact that lingering after intercourse without cleaning up can lead to what's coyly referred to as "honeymooner's disease" and is otherwise known as cystitis or your basic bladder infection, some women are just more fastidious than others. According to 28-year-old consultant Jennifer, "Getting clean first is important." Thirty-year-old designer Abbey is a little blunter: "I need to go clean up. I hate lingering in juices. Give me a damn tissue!" It's nothing personal, though. Jennifer, a 30-year-old banker, says, "Don't get mad if we want to shower and put our clothes on. Sometimes we just want to get comfortable before we snuggle."

Know That Once Might Not Be Enough

Cuddling? Not quite yet. Sleep? Not likely! At least not according to the hot-blooded women in our survey who aren't satisfied with one go-around. "I might want more," says Francesca, a 39-year-old education professional. Troy, a 29-year-old lawyer, wants men to know that "the woman isn't necessarily done just because they've fucked and he's come." Which brings us to another point: Sometimes, your job isn't over after you've climaxed. Your partner may need some more attention before she can even think about cuddling with you. "If you didn't make her come, you need to take care of that," says Bryn, a 41-year-old secretary.

But don't worry, gents. Not all women expect instantaneous response. "I might want to go again," says Elizabeth, a 28-year-old advertising sales manager, "but only when he's ready!"

If you're a one-shot kind of man (and most are, given the refractory period men need before they can have another erection), know that there are women who find it a turnoff when a man "expects seconds," in the words of Meagen, a 37-year-old psychotherapist. Bryn finds it really irritating after sex "when the man is suddenly interested in foreplay. WTF? Touch my breasts before, not after."

Here are a few more diverse thoughts about the postcoital period:

> "If I masturbate afterward, it doesn't mean he wasn't good enough. It means sex with him was *so* good that I want even more stimulation."
> **Carrie, 40, scientist**

> "I enjoy feeling his soft wet cock inside me for a time, and rubbing it against my pelvic floor. This will give me another orgasm, extending the experience."
> **Embe, 52, bodyworker**

> "It's a very honest time: If I'm in love, I want his attention. If I'm not really in love, I rather want my space then."
> **Sara, 30, engineer**

> "Women can be like the typical guy—after having sex, they're ready to move on to the next thing."
> **Carissa, 34, communications consultant**

> "I don't want to look dreamily into your eyes. I want to go to sleep or talk or do something normal. Maybe eat some food."
> **Ilea, 24, actuarial analyst**

> "If it's our first couple of times having sex together, our minds are racing and overthinking everything. Anything men can do to ease our overactive brains and make us feel comfortable and secure, the better. Make us laugh."
> **Summer, 27, TV advertising executive**

And for a very informative tidbit about how some women work, Judy, a 36-year-old teacher, lets us in on this little secret: "If I'm alert, it means I didn't orgasm. If I'm sleepy, I did."

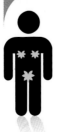

"It's a very honest time: If I'm in love, I want his attention."

Sara, 30, engineer

Ending a Bang with a Whimper: The Biggest After-Sex Turnoffs

We've told you what works for women after sex. Now let's talk about what *doesn't* work. We asked women to cite their biggest post-sex (or morning-after) turnoff or, in other words, what a guy can do to ensure there won't be a repeat performance.

Give Her the Cold Shoulder

According to the majority of our respondents, nothing says "jerk" like ignoring a woman when sex is over. You know, the "wham, bam, thank you ma'am" syndrome—but without even the courtesy of the "thank you ma'am." As Maureen, a 45-year-old archeologist, puts it, "I may not want the mushy stuff, but I don't want to feel like a used Kleenex, either. At least pretend you still want my company!"

Keite, a 31-year-old office manager, hates it "when a guy completely loses interest in any interaction with me whatsoever. Falling asleep is fine, whatever, but rolling over and turning out the light is not okay." Neither is "a total lack of interest when the deed is done," according to 46-year-old writer Inara.

Michelle, a 35-year-old marketing project manager, will give a guy the boot "if he completely disengages—as if I'm not there, or nothing just happened." Same with Sara, a 27-year-old CPA, who cites her biggest turnoff as a man "not being affectionate, pretending like last night didn't happen." And 27-year-old Summer, a TV advertising executive, says the worst behavior is not showing an ounce of romance or emotion. "I'm not saying that I need constant cuddling and roses," she says, "but a simple brush of the hair and even a quick arm around the waist goes a long way."

> "…a simple brush of the hair and even a quick arm around the waist goes a long way."
>
> **Summer, 27, TV advertising executive**

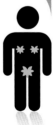

Basically, any drastic change in behavior or treatment from pre- to postcoitus is a huge warning sign to most women. Thirty-two-year-old business executive Suzy will walk away if a man acts "aloof, like now he's done with me." Maureen is turned off by "obvious disinterest in my company once my usefulness has ended." And Julie, a 43-year-old artist and writer, has definite reservations about a man who "seems embarrassed or unsure about what we did the night before."

According to Abbey, a 30-year-old designer, a man doesn't necessarily even have to act purposefully aloof to ruin the moment. All he has to do is "instantly go back to what he was doing without even a moment of relaxed enjoyment of what just happened." Let's face it, it's not very flattering to a woman when her partner acts remote—or asks for the remote—right after sex. When a man "immediately turns his attention to something else—TV, a book," it makes Sophie, a 45-year-old designer, "feel he's had it on his mind during sex."

Keep in mind, gentlemen, that this behavior is not limited to new relationships or one-night stands. Stacey, a 33-year-old marketing professional, still has problems "when my husband rolls over and faces the other side of the room. Feels like 'I'm done with you now.'"

So even if you're not feeling the love, guys, at least remember your manners long enough to let your partner feel good about having slept with you. A little goes a long way and can make the difference between a pleasantly memorable night and one she'd rather forget.

Do a "Hit and Run"

Leaving without saying goodbye is up there with pretending sex never happened or giving her the cold shoulder. Committing a "hit and run" is a direct and literal way for a man to distance himself physically and emotionally from his lover. It's sure to make a woman feel like the "used Kleenex" mentioned by Maureen.

"Rushing off to do something else like sex was a checkbox on a to-do list" really irritates project manager Ginger, 38. And 50-year-old Jackie checks a man off *her* list "if he runs for the door. Take me out to breakfast, for goodness sakes!" Twenty-nine-year-old performer Ulla tells us what she thinks is the rudest postcoital behavior: "Getting up and getting ready to leave. *His* apartment. To go to a party. And not inviting me. This actually happened." Ouch.

You don't actually have to even exit the building to give a woman that not-so-special feeling of having served her purpose. Leaving the bed, getting dressed right away, or running for the shower delivers the same message. Cari, a 26-year-old administrative assistant, can't stand it when a man feels the need to shimmy back into his jeans and shirt. "Chill out," she says. "No one's kicking you out right now!"

If you're interested in a woman and want, at the very least, another date, pay attention to your partner. Dawn, a 29-year-old PR executive, suggests, "Clue in to my needs. If I'm cuddling up to you, and talking about my hopes and dreams, don't turn on the TV or hop in the shower."

And actually, you don't even have to leave the bed to make her feel abandoned. "I hate when men pull out quickly," says 39-year-old Helena, a professor. "I'm happy to chat, fall asleep, etc., with him still inside me."

Last but not least, if you have a woman over to your place, try to avoid getting up and handing her clothes to her. "It says 'Get out, I'm done,'" says 44-year-old manager Annette. Of course, if that's the message you're trying to convey, it's your choice. But even if you're not interested in another encounter with the woman involved, it still makes you look like an asshole.

Criticize and Complain

Another way to crash and burn with a woman is to critique the sex after the fact. Remember, we're not talking the Olympics here, and no one cares what score the Russian judges—or you—give to her oral technique or how she uses her legs during lovemaking. It's rude and shows a lack of appreciation. Sarah, a 30-year-old salesperson, tells us, "I dated a guy who wanted to analyze the sex we just had. Every single time." We're wondering where the body's buried.

It's also bad form to "compare the sex you just had to other sexual experiences," says Karen, a 35-year-old student (along with many other women). If you can't imagine why this would bother someone, ask yourself how you'd feel if your partner, while lying there in the afterglow, said, "That was okay, but so-and-so used to go much longer . . . Oh, and he used his tongue completely differently, too."

We didn't think you'd like it. Not Caring About Appearance (Both Yours and Your Home's)

To some women, how much care a man takes with his grooming the morning after can also make a difference. According to Sara, a 30-year-old engineer, "If he doesn't care at all about his appearance after sex, I get the impression he just faked his good appearance to conquer me and get me into bed." So don't automatically stop shaving and break out your faded, holey T-shirts and ragged jeans just because you're sleeping with someone. Remember, just because you caught the bus once doesn't mean you won't have to do a little running to catch it next time.

"I hate when men pull out quickly"

Helena, 39, professor

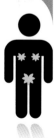

Good hygiene also extends to one's surroundings, so make an effort to straighten up if you're planning on having a woman over for a romantic interlude. Nothing says antiaphrodisiac like smelly socks and dirty underwear lying on the floor. We're not saying you have to go all Monk and straighten the edges of all your books and magazines so they match perfectly, but if you've got a collection of mold spores growing inside old pizza cartons, this would be a good time to abandon the science project and clean things up.

If you're a pet owner, remember that not everyone shares your fondness for cuddling with cats or dogs, at least not during or right after sex. Brianna, a 30-year-old marketing specialist, told us that her postcoital pet peeve (pun intended) is "having smelly dogs share the bed with us. Yuck." Saying "love me, love my dog" is all well and good, but there's a time and place for everything. Post-sex might not be the best time or place to include your pets.

Hooray for Sex!

Never forget that sex isn't just about achieving orgasm. It's about enjoyment and pleasure. It doesn't have to be a serious drama, and yes, it's okay to laugh while you're exploring each other's bodies and desires!

> "It's all about fun and play—let's indulge!"
> **Georgie, 43, editor**

> "I'm really satisfied at the moment. For me, it's really the greatest if my partner is open to exploring new things and we can discover each other together."
> **Matilda, 32, pharmacist**

How to Be Rude in Four Easy Steps

Different things piss off different women, but there are some basic behaviors you can bet most women will find off-putting, if not downright repugnant, after sex. If you know what's good for you, don't try any of the following.

Make Insensitive and Inappropriate Remarks

Rude remarks can be a real deal-killer after sex. Elizabeth, a 32-year-old mental health provider, finds it totally off-putting if a guy "says something insensitive to me or about others." And 45-year-old writer Roxanne has no patience for a man "if he's rude or mean in any way. It's a vulnerable moment."

By the way, talking about other women and past relationships, whether good or bad, definitely falls under the category of insensitive and inappropriate. Seraphin, a 40-year-old technology strategist, tells us that her ex "wasn't quite over some of his past relationships," which at least partially explains why he's her ex now. The last thing a woman wants to hear is anything about other women right after a man has made love to *her*. Says Rachel, 45, an entrepreneur, "Don't talk about other sexual partners during this time. EVER!!!" It seems obvious, but evidently there are men out there who don't understand why a comment like "You have nice breasts. Of course, they're not as big as my last girlfriend's, but I like smaller breasts anyway," might be a little offensive. A remark doesn't have to be that obvious to cast a damper over the afterglow. If you're comparison shopping, keep it to yourself.

> **"Don't talk about other sexual partners during this time. EVER!!!"**
>
> **Rachel, 45, entrepreneur**

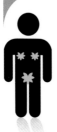

Answer the Phone. During Sex.

Don't answer the phone when you're getting intimate with someone. We can't quite believe we have to point this out, but apparently we do, judging from some of the comments we read from our survey respondents. Katherine, a 38-year-old manager, finds it totally off-putting "when another girl calls" when she's with a man (and he answers). Not surprisingly, guys that "answer the phone during sex" win no points with 55-year-old Paula and a host of other women. Several women also commented that picking up the phone or initiating a call *after* sex is a surefire way to get a "thanks, but no thanks" when you ask for another date. Unless you're a brain surgeon or have some other profession where lives may depend on you picking up a call, let it go to voice mail.

Pass Gas

Although some people find fart jokes hilarious, several women in our survey said they don't find farting funny, attractive, or appropriate after (or during) sex. Leave Terrance and Philip at home, gents, unless you're sure your gal is the sort who delights in pulling your finger when dared. Now, this isn't to say that an accidental release of gas is a deal-breaker. Men often express relief when they're taken off "fart hold," that period early in a relationship where you don't dare pass gas in her presence. That doesn't mean, however, that it's time for letting it rip under the covers and giving her a Dutch oven. Be nice.

Snoring is also on the hit list, but that's not always under a man's (or a woman's) control. If you know you have a habit of sawing logs when asleep, at least issue fair warning and maybe a pair of earplugs.

Commit Any of These Miscellaneous Maneuvers

Here are just a few other things that turn a happy postcoital session into a postmortem for the relationship. Women really despise it when guys:

"Talk about daily things, chores, work, etc."
Vanessa, 35, administrator

"Thank me. Like it was something I had to do. What's up with that?"
Jane, 39, businesswoman (We guess there is such a thing as being too polite.)

"Get too clingy or butch."
Jyllian, 44, engineer, mom

"Go crazy with the 'love' talk."
Ilea, 24, actuarial analyst

"Ask the question: 'Did you come?'"
Matilda, 32, pharmacist

"Tell her that he 'Supermanned that ho.'"
Leslie, 30, national account specialist
(Translation: ejaculating on a woman's back so that the sheet sticks to her like 'Superman's cape'—thank you, Urban Dictionary!)

"Come all over himself and then rub up on me. Talk about his mother or meeting his family. Tell me the condom broke. Say 'I feel a cold sore coming on.' Or 'I have to put my roommate's toy back before he/she gets home.' Do I need to give more real-life examples?"
Grape, 32, model/actress

Nope, we get the picture!

The Bottom Line

We hope that what you've picked up from this chapter is that a little sensitivity goes a long way during the after-sex period. It all comes down to this: Treat her like you'd like to be treated. Don't be a jerk, in other words. Kiss her, tell her how great she was, snuggle up, and enjoy the afterglow.

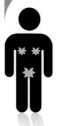

"It's all about fun and play— let's indulge!"

Georgie, 43, editor

Chapter 8

Flights of Fancy

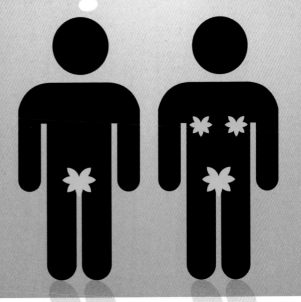

Sexual fantasies play a definite role in the feminine psyche. Women just don't always talk about it. So we asked our survey takers to tell us about their fantasies: whether or not they had them, what they were about, and whether they were interested in sharing them with a lover. The responses (par for the course) blew us away.

"My fantasies are far stranger than you'd ever imagine."

Jyllian, 44, engineer, mom

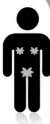

What Women Wish Men Knew about Their Sexual Fantasies

What do women wish you knew about their fantasies? First and foremost, they have them! Lots of them. They may not always want to share their fantasies with their partners (although many of them do, and we'll get to that!), but, as Judy, a 59-year-old clinical researcher, puts it, "I have them as often as they do." Fantasies let women take charge of their sexuality and re-create themselves within the confines of the bedroom . . . or wherever they choose to play. "I want to feel feminine, sexy, and powerful," says Sam, a 35-year-old lawyer, in describing the role that her fantasies play for her.

So what do you need to know about your gal's inner life? Read on.

Women Fantasize About Sex—a Lot!

Fantasies are a part of life, running the gamut from gentle daydreams of the proverbial white knight in shining armor to hard-core erotic scenarios involving multiple partners, handcuffs, and candle wax. Anything and everything. The imagination is a powerful tool for women when it comes to creating sexual tension and/or providing stimulus to reach orgasm. You never know what goes on behind those demure (or not so demure) exteriors. As 37-year-old marine biologist Heather confesses, her fantasies "are probably just as dirty, if not dirtier, than yours."

"I have fantasies," says Michelle, a 36-year-old management consultant. "A conservative exterior doesn't mean a prudish interior!" And Michelle is not the only one. Forty-year-old travel writer Shannon tells us, "Just because I'm a nice Midwestern girl doesn't mean I don't have any fantasies. I'm open to trying things." Abbey, a 30-year-old designer, says her fantasies are "vivid and they are many."

Don't Be Threatened by Her Fantasies (Especially If They're Not about You)

Don't worry. You're not being replaced by a phantom hottie. "Fantasizing," 32-year-old Alli assures us, "doesn't mean I'm not into him." Fantasies are not a substitute for the act of sex, but rather an enhancement to the experience. Says Monica, a 49-year-old restaurant owner, "They (fantasies) don't lesson our desire for our partner. Talking about fantasies without being defensive can be great foreplay."

You may even be in them. "The fantasies don't always include celebrities and random strangers," points out 27-year-old Summer, an advertising executive. "A lot of the time the fantasy includes *you*, so take advantage and make them a reality."

And if they're not about you, no big deal, either. Just as men enjoy looking at *Playboy* (yes, it's all about the articles . . . that's the ticket!), a lot of women get their engines revved by fantasizing about celebrities, characters in books or movies, and even faceless men or women. When asked about her fantasies, 29-year-old lawyer Troy confesses, "They involve men other than a partner." And Carrie, a 40-year-old scientist, admits that her partner is "probably not in my fantasies. Men should probably not know that unless they can get in touch with Richard Gere from *Pretty Woman* and have him play the piano. Or Pierce Brosnan." Domestic executive Dawn, 42, tells us, "I just have a lot of sex with rock stars, like Roger Daltry, and actors. Like Brad Pitt—but only in *Snatch*."

Let's face it. Some women are not comfortable mixing their fantasies with their real-life partners. "I would love to have sex with multiple male and female partners," Kelly, a 32-year-old wildlife biologist, tells us, "but not if my fiancé is one of them." If he's lucky, maybe Kelly will let her fiancé watch.

Have No Fear

This is part of the whole "every woman is different" lesson we're trying to impart here. It's important to remember (which is why we keep reiterating this point) that even if you spent ten years with one woman and had her sexual preferences down to a fine art, the next woman you sleep with may have diametrically opposed likes and dislikes. Imagine yourself as Captain Kirk, exploring strange new worlds, seeking out new G-spots and different sexual preferences . . . boldly going where . . . well, we'll let our respondents say a few words here:

> "Every person and every moment is different. Don't be afraid to try new things. If they don't work, it's okay. We're all human, and women appreciate the effort."
> **Ilea, 24, actuarial analyst**

> "Enthusiasm goes a long way! Confidence and experimentation also. I think sex can be a spiritual experience, but few men seem to feel that way or want to explore it."
> **Beth, 43, designer**

Don't Worry: Fantasy Doesn't Always Equal Reality

Just because women have fantasies doesn't mean that they're interested in acting them out. "Fantasies are mostly just fun to talk about," says 36-year-old astrologer Ursula. Lula, a 30-year-old librarian, agrees. "I don't always want to make my fantasies a reality," she says. And 43-year-old artist/writer Julie has this to say: "Fantasy isn't the same as reality—it's fun to play, but it doesn't reflect the desire for something to happen in real life."

Why? Women gave different reasons for wanting their fantasies to remain in the realm of their imagination. Sometimes it's because they're not comfortable with bringing hidden desires into the light of day. "They're not always PC," says Sophie, a 45-year-old designer, about her fantasies, "and they should be kept separate from public life." Jackie, a 50-year-old artist, admits, "Most of my sexual fantasies are nothing I would ever consider doing in real life." Michelle, a 35-year-old marketing project manager, states unequivocally, "They are fantasies, and I don't really ever want them to come true."

Like we said, some women use their fantasies as a way to rev up the sexual engines. Forty-five-year-old writer Roxanne puts it this way, "Just because I have a certain fantasy doesn't mean I want to try it. It's just my 'go-to' mental method for getting myself turned on." Domestic executive Dawn agrees. "It's just a mental thing," she says. "It's nothing I'd actually want to do."

Others like to keep their fantasies and actual sex life separate because they don't want their fantasies spoiled if a real-life enactment

> **"Fantasy isn't the same as reality— it's fun to play, but it doesn't reflect the desire for something to happen in real life."**
>
> Julie, 43, artist/writer

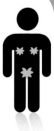

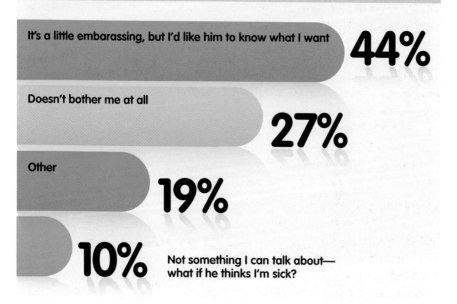

How comfortable are you sharing your fantasies with your lover?

It's a little embarrassing, but I'd like him to know what I want **44%**

Doesn't bother me at all **27%**

Other **19%**

10% Not something I can talk about—what if he thinks I'm sick?

Note: Percentages may not equal 100% due to rounding.

falls short of their imagination. As Nara, a 41-year-old massage therapist, puts it (perhaps from experience): "Reality is rarely as good as fantasy."

She May Be Shy about Sharing Her Fantasies

We asked our survey respondents whether or not they were comfortable sharing their fantasies with their partners. The answer? The majority of women are a little embarrassed, but willing to deal with it to let their guys (or gals) know what they want. Quite a few expressed a willingness to share if their partners expressed an interest in the subject. To quote Sara, a 27-year-old CPA: "I'm more willing to share if you ask." Forty-year-old administrative manager Andrea urges men to "keep asking questions—be sensitive and respectful, but I want you to encourage me to share my fantasies." And the majority of these women feel it would be in the man's best interest to learn about their innermost desires. "I'm open to trying almost anything," says Nana, a 37-year-old marketing manager. "Just ask."

A smaller percentage—about 27 percent—don't mind talking about their fantasies one bit. In fact, "just talking about them turns me on!" says Cari, a 26-year-old administrative assistant. Thirty-two-year-old Christina, who works in marketing and advertising, wants men to know that "we have fantasies, and they should be explored. Communication has to happen." And Adrianna, a 33-year-old household engineer, shares her fantasies *because* she wants to enact them: "When we tell you about our fantasies, help us fulfill them in the way we describe them."

However, if you expect your partner to open up, be prepared to respond in kind. Although there are some women (and men) who prefer to monologue their way through life, most people aren't comfortable sharing their innermost thoughts if their partner keeps theirs hidden. As Karren, a 45-year-old attorney, puts it, "I don't mind sharing, but I want reciprocity."

Ten percent of the women we surveyed aren't interested in exposing their fantasies at all. "I don't want them to know," states Breanna, a 51-year-old in the publishing industry. "Then it's not my fantasy." And 30-year-old attorney Emily definitely prefers to keep hers secret. "I'm happy for them to think I'm thinking about sweet girl things," she says. Troy, a 29-year-old lawyer, has this to say about her fantasies: "They are shallow and private and unimportant to anyone other than me."

Sometimes women are unwilling to share for fear of what their partners might think of them. Says 41-year-old secretary Bryn, "Not every sexual fantasy is fit to be shared. I don't have pleasant little fantasies about him or role-playing. Most of my fantasies are rough and violent, and are not necessarily anything I'd want to play out with him."

> **"A lot of my fantasies are for me alone."**
>
> Abbey, 30, designer

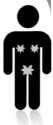

So what's a man to do? You might share one of your tamer fantasies with her, to see whether it sparks anything. But if she's reluctant to reciprocate, don't push. And if she *does* share a shocking fantasy, for God's sake, don't react negatively. Remember that it's called a fantasy for a reason.

Sharing Is Situational

For some women, as with most issues to do with seduction, foreplay, and sex, their willingness to open up about their secret desires "depends on the partner." According to management consultant Michelle, "With my current partner, we tell each other our fantasies. It's fun. I didn't with my last long-term partner. It just didn't seem like something he'd appreciate." As for 40-year-old technology strategist Seraphin, it all depends on whether she's looking at the long term or not—and surprisingly, the more serious she is about a guy, the less willing she is to open up. "If I really think we have a future together," she says, "I don't want to talk about them with him."

Some women just aren't interested in sharing, period. "It doesn't bother me," shrugs Troy, "but I rarely share them. It's a fantasy, and I don't want it to be much more than what it is: a masturbation aid." She's not the only one. "A lot of my fantasies are for me alone," states Abbey, a 30-year-old designer. "I use them for masturbating." Marketing project manager Michelle thinks that "fantasies are for the person having them. There's no point in sharing."

And Sometimes Reality Is SO Good . . .

Not all women want or need fantasies if their partner is doing the job for them. Marla, a 44-year-old singer, has this to say about her man: "He does such a good job that I don't really fantasize." Sylvia, a 48-year-old marketing rep, says that "if we have a good relationship, inside and outside the bedroom, I don't really think about fantasies."

Guys, *please* don't take this to mean that her fantasies are an indication that you don't measure up. On the contrary. A vivid sexual fantasy life may mean that you keep her engines purring constantly. Again, it all depends on the woman.

What Is She Fantasizing About?

So given that women fantasize, what are they fantasizing about? The only way you're going to find out what *your* woman fantasizes is by asking her. That much became clear when we asked our survey respondents to share the topics of their erotic daydreams. There are definitely common themes running through the feminine psyche: Many women enjoy benevolent manhandling, for instance—things like having their wrists pinned to the bed, having their partner grab their hair while kissing them, or having control taken away to some extent. But some of the fantasies expressed by our survey respondents are, to say the least, unique. Remember what we said about "everything and anything"? We really weren't kidding.

Her Fantasies Are All Over the Map

Think you've got a good idea what your gal's daydreaming about? Not so fast. One of the things we found out from our survey results is just how varied women's fantasies can be. Here's a sampling:

"Spontaneous behavior, like throwing me on the kitchen table and kissing me all over." And "Blindfolding me and using a feather all over."
Arianna, 33, household engineer

"I love to be out in nature, and if there are other people nearby that might hear us . . . well, that's even more of a turn-on."
Embe, 52, bodyworker

"I'm a submissive hooker who gets turned on despite her intentions not to."
Marisol, 66, writer

"I get off on fantasizing about Michelangelo's statues come to life."
Taylor, 65, comedy writer

"Dressing up in sexy clothes and stripping."
January, 47, paralegal

Here's the winner for the "Can't Pick Just One" award:

"I'd say a sprinkling of everything, with the exception of things involving pain. Something as simple as fantasizing about sex with a person I'm interested in can do it, or wilder things, including (but not limited to) sex in public places, casual sex, three- or moresomes, lesbian/gay, dominance/submission, prostitution/performance, bestiality, age difference, etc."
Mae, 31, graduate student

And the winner for most unique fantasy:

"What I call the 'Armageddon fuck.' The sort of fuck that you wouldn't want to have to wake up in the morning and face the guy you did it with. Either because the act is too far gone or because the

fantasy guy is too revolting. Hence, only the kind of sex you'd want to have if the world were coming to an end."
Bryn, 41, secretary

Just goes to show there really is something for everybody.

Her Fantasies Might Be Fairly Tame
Not everyone has wild, elaborate role-playing in mind when they fantasize. For instance, 24-year-old actuarial analyst Ilea says that her fantasies "don't need to be crazy, but just keep it interesting." And Adrienne, a 33-year-old masters student, tells us her fantasies are definitely "not over-the-top. Just the two of us, naked, having a great time."

Romance, as opposed to whips and chains, is what turns some women on. "My fantasies are pretty tame," says Rose, a 30-year-old teacher. "I mostly want to be with my partner in a fantastically romantic setting and for us to just be in the moment."

So make it romantic and make sure your mind is on your partner, and *not* on work or the Super Bowl, no matter *how* good the commercials might be!

Sometimes It's about Her. And Her.
We know this couldn't *possibly* be of interest to most men (yes, we're lying), but sometimes women are turned on by the thought of having sex with other women, whether or not they'd follow through in real life. When asked about her erotic wish list, Kate, a 34-year-old physician, confesses that some of them "often involve other women." Although Faith, a 25-year-old who works in sales, maintains that "fantasizing about girls does not make you a lesbian," it's still something that turns her on. Seventy-year-old writer Wendy doesn't equivocate and states bluntly: "Lesbian sex is a turn-on."

> **"I mostly want to be with my partner in a fantastically romantic setting and for us to just be in the moment."**
>
> **Rose, 30, teacher**

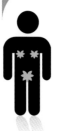

Yes, She Thinks about Threesomes

It's a standard stereotype that guys are totally into the idea of threesomes (usually involving themselves and two smoking-hot lesbians who just happen to have the hots for the guy, too), but it may come as a surprise that some women also have fantasies involving more than one person. Not all, mind you. For some women, the idea of sharing their man with either another male or another female is on their list of turnoffs. But others, like Dawn, a 29-year-old public relations executive, find the thought of a threesome as much of a turn-on as you might. "We think about having threesomes and having a wild one-night stand as much as men do," she says. Confesses 36-year-old physician Liz, "I would like to have a threesome . . . sex with two men and sex with a man and a woman."

Forty-five-year-old writer Roxanne admits to spending time "fantasizing about being in a threesome (two men, one woman), or being 'shared' by multiple men." And Karren, a 45-year-old attorney, takes the threesome idea up a notch and is turned on by the thought of "being blindfolded with multiple people touching me."

Keep in mind that even though your partner may enjoy the thought of having sex with more than one person at a time, it's not always something she wants to do in real life. Matilda, a 32-year-old pharmacist, is very clear that "in my case, they *are* fantasies. I can, for example, have a fantasy of a threesome with another woman but it does not mean that I actually want to do it."

> **"We think about having three- somes and having a wild one-night stand as much as men do."**
>
> **Dawn, public relations executive**

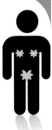

Have you ever taken a picture of, or videotaped, yourself having sex?

NO **65%**

YES **35%**

Note: Percentages may not equal 100% due to rounding.

She Fantasizes About Being Watched

There's a reason reality shows are so popular these days. People have a strong streak of voyeurism, and sometimes this extends to the bedroom. Take Caroline, a 29-year-old teacher, for instance, who's turned on by "the idea that his friends or his bandmates are watching us have sex, and possibly waiting to take a turn with me." Or management consultant Michelle, who enjoys "fantasies where other people are watching us." Pat, a 56-year-old project manager, loves to think about "my lover watching while I get it on with another man." Twenty-five-year-old administrator Vanessa is titillated by thought of "being caught masturbating."

So how many women have actually begun to enact this fantasy by letting their partners take pictures or videotape them during sex? Only about 35 percent, according to our survey. The rest, no doubt cognizant of the dangers of YouTube, keep the camera turned off.

Let the Games Begin

Just as someone who's shy in everyday life can be a total ham on stage, it's often easier for people to lose themselves in a fantasy scenario if they are not "playing" themselves. Give some gals a costume and it can open up aspects of themselves they don't usually let out. Clothes can play a huge part in this transformation. "Picture a Halloween party," says Judy. "If there's a costume, I'm there." Julie, a 43-year-old artist and writer, likes "historical scenarios," and Alex, a 35-year-old college professor, prefers "period costumes and situations."

So we asked our survey respondents what they thought about role-playing games with their lovers.

The majority—nearly 45 percent—of the women we questioned are into it if they're in the right mood and it's the right partner,

while 35 percent have never tried it. About 9 percent have tried it and have no interest in repeating the experience. For librarian Lulu, it's very simple: "I don't like having to act a part. I feel stupid, not sexy."

For those women who are either all for trying it again or could be convinced to play under the right circumstances, it helps if they feel safe and taken seriously by their partners—not just that you're humoring them. Heather, a 28-year-old travel photographer, says, "I have to feel supported and comfortable, and then things could get exceptional."

Costumes don't always factor into role-playing, by the way. Sometimes it can be as simple as pretending to be someone you're not. Here's a sampler of the scenarios women have:

> "The office fantasy (boss/secretary), the doctor's office fantasy (doctor/patient). I think I'm naturally more of a submissive." **Sunny, 36, project manager**

"I have to feel supported and comfortable, and then things could get exceptional."

Heather, travel photographer

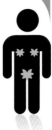

What do you think about role-playing/fantasy games with your partner?

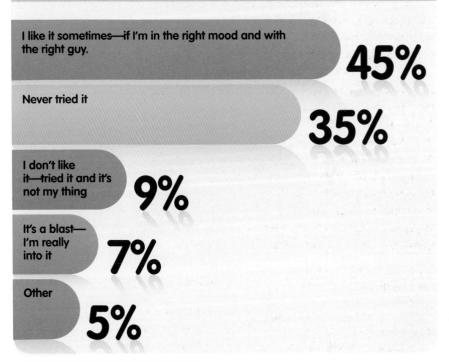

I like it sometimes—if I'm in the right mood and with the right guy. 45%

Never tried it 35%

I don't like it—tried it and it's not my thing 9%

It's a blast—I'm really into it 7%

Other 5%

Note: Percentages may not equal 100% due to rounding.

"Uniforms and housewives, business execs and secretary."
Leilani, 31, pharmaceutical sales

"I'm really into the idea of boss/secretary role-play right now."
Ellen, 32, Web development team manager

"Schoolgirl/teacher."
Kate, 35, writer

"Rock 'n roll fantasies, movie scenes."
Rachel, 45, entrepreneur

"Usually forbidden situations like boss/secretary, maid/homeowner."
Keite, 31, office manager

"Being a hooker."
Marisol, 66, writer

"Having sex with a stranger in a public place."
Frankie, 36, swim instructor

Odds are if you ask your partner about assuming a different role in bed, show genuine interest in her ideas, and don't laugh at her reply, you can be assured of some interesting and sexy games.

Not Her Game

Which fantasies or role-playing games are women *least* turned on by? In other words, what are their personal taboos?

Bodily Functions

Heading the list is anything to do with bodily functions. "Bodily functions and humiliation fantasies are icky," says Rachel, 45, an entrepreneur. In fact, most of the women we surveyed find fantasies involving bodily fluids repugnant, especially when they're joined with humiliation scenarios. Thirty-year-old project manager Ginger states that "things that demean or humiliate are mental issues I'm not into."

On the list of "not for me" for many women, including 32-year-old actress Grape, are "golden showers, or glass bottom boat—no thank you." Forty-six-year-old writer Inara wants "nothing to do with urine, feces, or diapers." Julie ups the ante of "no way!" fantasies with her list of "anything to do with excrement, animals, or children."

Sometimes the definition of bodily fluids extends to your manly essence. Sorry, guys, but no matter what they show in some of your favorite XXX flicks, not every woman gets off on having a man ejaculate on her face. Marla, a 30-year-old artist, doesn't (sorry about this) make any bones about the fact that "I don't like to have him jack off on my face."

Rape Fantasies

Although a scenario involving being overpowered figures in many women's fantasies, they draw the line at enacting them, and to some women, these thoughts are in fact the very opposite of erotic. "Rape fantasies are a big turnoff" for attorney Karren, 45. She's not the only one. Writer Kate, 35, tells us, "One guy wanted to try a rape scenario, and I said, 'No way.'" And even if a woman is into a rape scenario, "men should be aware that's something that should ALWAYS be initiated by a woman, on general principles," Troy cautions.

Bottom line here, gents, is that if you want to play out a nonconsensual fantasy with your lover, make sure it's a consensual choice.

Anal Sex

Speaking of the bottom line (sorry, sorry . . . but could you resist it? Didn't think so!), some women find the thought of anal sex or anything to do with the flip side of genitalia a total turnoff. Maureen, our archeologist, says, "Anal sex is not attractive to me," and her stance is echoed by many—though not all—of our survey respondents. "I'm NOT licking your ass," Caroline states firmly. Meagen, a 37-year-old psychotherapist, has similar feelings on the subject. "He wanted me to lick his anus," she recalls of a past lover. "Sorry, but my tongue does not go there."

Threesomes

Even though some women are totally into the idea of threesomes, for others, three (or more) is definitely a crowd when it comes to sex. "I don't want to share," says Annette, a 44-year-old manager. For some women, it's an issue of feeling they're not enough for their lover. Grad student Melanie says, "Repeated threesome fantasies make me feel inadequate on my own."

Feeling Left Out

Other women dislike fantasies where they feel they're not really included. Emily, a 30-year-old attorney, doesn't care for a guy "asking me to pretend to be something I'm clearly not. I think he's not really into me." Thirty-eight-year-old manager Katherine finds it very off-putting to be in the middle of a sexual encounter "when you suddenly realize there is no resemblance of 'you' in the picture!"

Other turnoffs include (but are not limited to):

"My lover wanting me to get it on with another woman. Sorry, just not my thing."
Pat, 56, project manager

"Pretend that I am gay."
Leslie, 30, national account specialist

"Man with another man."
Mallory, 28, mother

"Anything that has to do with being younger than 18."
Georgie, 43, editor

"Little girl/daddy fantasy."
Roxy, 31, administrator

"A boyfriend once confessed that he had worn a pair of my thong underwear while masturbating. That was the beginning of the end."
Roxanne, 45, writer

"Oral sex in costume."
Taylor, 35, teacher

And the winner for longest list of sexual no-no's:

"Wearing a strap-on and taking him up the ass, wearing B&D gear that most certainly other exes had also worn or used. Also, although I've never been asked to do any of these: anything having to do with excrement, blood, violence, extreme B&D, humiliation, Saran wrap, electricity."
Seraphin, 40, technology strategist

Toy Time

Adult toys like vibrators and dildos can play an important part in a couple's sex life, whether indulging in fantasies or just augmenting daily "vanilla" lovemaking. Although these props have become more mainstream thanks to shows like *Sex and the City*, we wondered whether women find it embarrassing to have their guy (or gal) help pick them out. So of course we asked them. The results? Nearly 75 percent of our respondents said they'd "love it" if their lover joined them in picking out their toys. "We always go together," says domestic executive Dawn. Judy says that she and her lover put an adult store on the itinerary every time they visit a new town. "It's part of the fun of travel!" she exclaims. Others use their shopping trip as an opportunity to get to know each other better. "It's fun to see what each of us wanders toward," says Annette.

A few women confessed to mixed emotions. "I'd feel slightly embarrassed, but also slightly turned on," said Sunny. And entrepreneur Rachel says that she'd have "more fun with a girl, but I don't mind with a guy." Others said it all depended on the guy.

Only about 6 percent wouldn't check out their local Good Vibrations with their dude. "I'd rather he just bring me toys," says Sarah, a 47-year-old attorney.

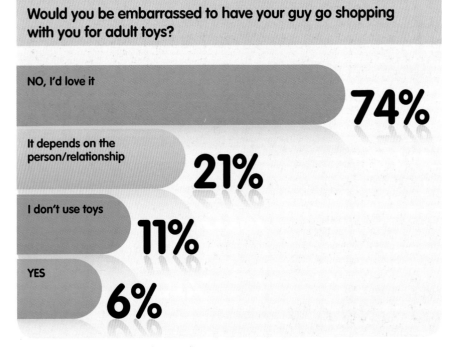

Would you be embarrassed to have your guy go shopping with you for adult toys?

NO, I'd love it — **74%**

It depends on the person/relationship — **21%**

I don't use toys — **11%**

YES — **6%**

Note: Percentages may not equal 100% due to rounding.

The Pornography Question

Guys, we know that most of you like pornography. As Cynthia confirmed in *What Men Really Want in Bed*, porn is a staple of the male sexual psyche. But most men also emphasize that women shouldn't be threatened by it. But are they? Yes and no.

About 27 percent of our survey respondents couldn't care less if you enjoy porn. "I'm glad he does," says Carrie, 40, a scientist. "He's sexually self-sufficient, and I'm never pressured to put out." In fact, the largest portion—34 percent—of the women we surveyed don't mind if their guy reads or looks at porn, on one condition: They want you to share! Pharmacist Matilda, for example, enjoys it as much as her man. "I like to read and watch it too, sometimes," she says. "It can be a turn-on for later." Seraphin also sees the upside to it: "Sex while watching or looking at porn can be quite hot." For 62-year-old Annie, a writer, "It depends on what kind of porn. Anything sadomasochistic is out. But some porn can be a turn-on and it wouldn't bother me to share it with him or let him watch it alone if he has to." Yet Annie went on to reflect a common concern

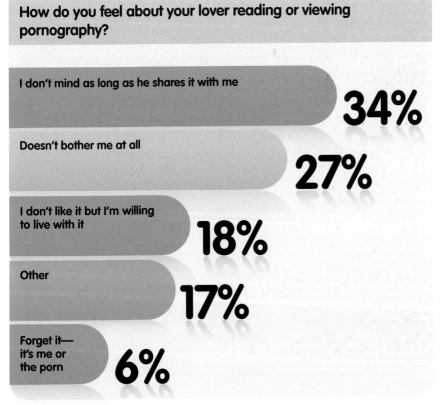

How do you feel about your lover reading or viewing pornography?

I don't mind as long as he shares it with me	**34%**
Doesn't bother me at all	**27%**
I don't like it but I'm willing to live with it	**18%**
Other	**17%**
Forget it—it's me or the porn	**6%**

Note: Percentages may not equal 100% due to rounding.

women have about porn: "I think I'd feel insecure about the women, though, because many of them are younger and in better shape than I am."

Sharing Porn—in Moderation

In fact, if he's going to look at it, women want their man to bring it out in the open. Secrecy is an issue, as swim instructor Frankie, 36, reports: "We look at it together . . . I wouldn't like it if he did it in secret, and often." Michelle, a management consultant, agrees that clandestine porn viewing can be problematic: "It depends on the guy," she says. "With my current partner, I wouldn't mind at all. With some guys, it might matter because they might be using it to suppress something else, or try to hide it. There's no need to hide it." But like most things,

pornography is fine as long as their guy consumes it in moderation. "It doesn't bother me as long as it's not excessive," says January, in a typical comment. How do you know when it's too much? If it's replacing the real thing, for one. "I don't mind at all as long as I'm the recipient of the lust," says Annette. "If it becomes a replacement for me, then it's got to go." As far as Ginger is concerned, porn "should be a nonissue if our sex life is meeting both our needs adequately."

For about 18 percent of the women we surveyed, it all depends—they'll live with it if they have to, but they're not crazy about it. Troy, for example, doesn't care if casual partners look at porn; however, she'd "dislike it strongly in someone I love or am in a relationship with, even if it's an open

"Sometimes I get curious and I watch Internet videos, but it makes me feel gross afterward."

Emily, 30, attorney

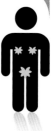

relationship. I dislike porn for political reasons, not because I think there's anything inherently wrong with the concept of watching people fuck." Bryn says, "I go through cycles. My husband's graduate school thesis is on porn, so sometimes I accept that he does look at a lot of it, but I really don't think that it's helpful to our marriage."

The A-word (as in "addiction") is the line in the sand for several women. Shai, a 33-year-old marketer, says, "I don't mind as long as 1) he doesn't need to watch it every time we have sex, and 2) he isn't addicted to it. In other words, occasional watching is okay, but watching every day is not okay." Kelly, a 32-year-old wildlife biologist and dance instructor, thinks porn "can be exciting, but it concerns me if it becomes a regular part of his life."

¡Erotica, Si! ¡Porn, No!

So if women have such mixed feelings about their guys looking at porn, do they look at it themselves? For slightly more than half of our respondents, the answer was "It depends." Women make a distinction between pornography and "erotica." Someday we'll ask them to explain the difference between the two, but based on the comments we got, it seems that "erotica" distinguishes itself in terms of its literary quality. In contrast, women described porn with terms like "humorous," "cheesy," and "boring."

"There are some fantastic erotic stories out there, but most porn leaves me fairly 'eh.' The movies make me giggle," says Inara, a 46-year-old writer. Marketing rep Sylvia, 48, says, "I've read some fiction that will put me in the mood, but I haven't deliberately read erotica to add to my pleasure. Porn movies leave me cold."

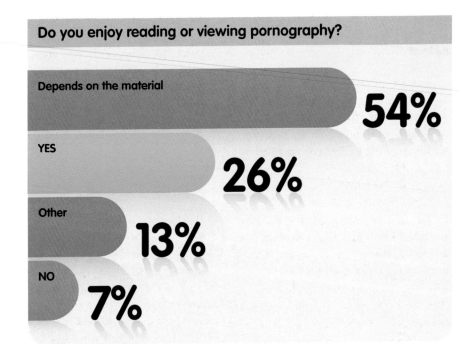

Do you enjoy reading or viewing pornography?

Depends on the material — **54%**

YES — **26%**

Other — **13%**

NO — **7%**

Note: Percentages may not equal 100% due to rounding.

Others are more open to it, depending on the partner and the circumstances. For scientist Carrie, it "depends on the material and the mood. Sometimes it's fun." Shannon, a 40-year-old travel writer, "wouldn't mind trying it with the right guy."

For several respondents, porn is a bit of a guilty pleasure. "I like it, but sometimes it makes me feel guilty because it's an exploitive industry," confesses Sam, while Emily, 30, says, "Sometimes I get curious and I watch Internet videos, but it makes me feel gross afterward." And Annette, a 44-year-old manager, is quite particular in her tastes: "I only like real lesbian porn, not straight girl-on-girl porn or guy-girl porn. Yes, you can tell the difference. Real lesbians kiss a lot more."

For a small percentage of our respondents, porn just doesn't do it for them at all. Singer Marla shrugs it off with "I don't see the need," and Ginger isn't really into it "because porn deals with the physical, and sex for me is often more mental."

Tie Me Up, Tie Me Down: BDSM

BDSM (bondage and discipline, domination and submission, and sadomasochism) has, to a certain extent, gone mainstream. For example, light bondage is no longer really seen as a fringe activity, as anyone who's seen prime-time TV shows like *Desperate Housewives* or *Mad Men* knows. So how do women really feel about walking on the wild side? As evidenced by some of the fantasies they shared, quite a few women find the thought of dominance/submission play and bondage quite titillating, provided it's all in fun and pain isn't a part of it. But when it comes to the harder stuff, nearly half said that it's not a place they want to go.

Thirty-year-old Sarah says, "I had a boyfriend who was into it, but I realized it wasn't for me. It never did it for me the way it did it for him. I found it boring." And Cari is "totally not into the S&M stuff, like choking or whipping hard, etc." Sam says, "It's not my thing, but I don't have a problem with other consenting adults doing it."

Others are open to it, within limits: 22 percent said that it all depends on the person and situation, while 18 percent are fine with BDSM as long as no one gets hurts. In other words, women's interest in BDSM is all a matter of degree. For example, when questioned directly about BSDM, 46-year-old writer Inara responds, "Leave out the pain part, but the rest is fun! Just leave the nipple clamps at home!" These women might explore a little "lighthearted" BDSM (if such a term can be

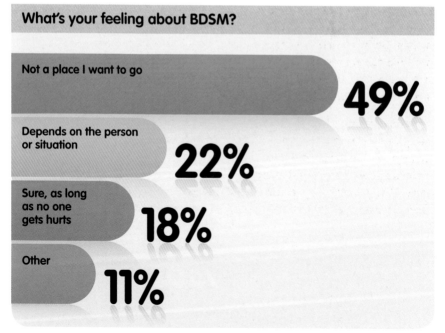

What's your feeling about BDSM?

Not a place I want to go — **49%**

Depends on the person or situation — **22%**

Sure, as long as no one gets hurts — **18%**

Other — **11%**

Note: *Percentages may not equal 100% due to rounding.*

used), but don't want to go too far. "I've experimented a little," 27-year-old lawyer Troy tells us. "I'm not into it and would stay away from men who are strongly into it, but I don't mind it experimentally to mix things up."

Bondage

A little light bondage? No big deal. At least, that's how it appears from the comments we got from our survey respondents. Helena, a 39-year-old professor, shares, "I like domination and direction, some tying up, blindfold kind of stuff, but probably pretty tame." And executive assistant Heather likes to indulge in "some light BDSM, but I'm more playful than super serious about it." Jenny, a 28-year-old medical office manager, on the other hand, says, "I like to be mastered, tied up, and blindfolded."

Then there are the gals who'd rather be on the other end of the rope, so to speak. Management consultant Michelle has "fantasies where I tie him up." And attorney Karren gets turned on thinking about "tying him up and teasing him for extended periods of time."

Again, it's all a matter of degree. Seraphin says, "Some very, very light bondage (holding arms back, aggressiveness, blindfolds) is fun sometimes, but anything other than that is disturbing, especially if he collects books about it and gets excited about new knots and configurations."

> **"Leave out the pain part, but the rest is fun! Just leave the nipple clamps at home!"**
>
> **Inara, 46, writer**

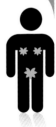

Domination

It's also a matter of degree and context when you're talking about domination and submission, which figures in the fantasies of many women who answered our survey. We think that this is because many gals spend their days trying to stay in control of every aspect of their lives, from their careers to their personal lives. It's an exhausting task, so it's no wonder they fantasize about letting go and being dominated in the bedroom. Inara, a 46-year-old writer, puts it like this: "I love being tied up and dominated, and anything that goes with that. It's just I'm such a control freak in my everyday life, I like to give up control in bed." And she's not the only one. "I wish more men were comfortable with taking a dominant stance," says Keite. "I enjoy being dominated," admits Ginger. "It makes me feel feminine." And Beth, a 43-year-old designer, likes "to have control taken away from me. But he has to be into it." (What this all says about gender roles could fill a doctoral thesis, and probably has.)

With some women, it goes beyond domination and into the realm of rough play. "Being a bit aggressive can turn me on," 34-year-old scientist Sisley tells us. Sara, a 30-year-old engineer, confesses, "I like it rough sometimes. Surprise me. Slam me up against a wall and rape me." Just don't get carried away with the caveman routine out of the bedroom, guys. What can turn a woman on during sex can really piss her off in any other context. As Sara clarifies, "I like being dominated, but only in bed."

Some women are very much into the entire BSDM scene. Jyllian, a 44-year-old engineer, admits to being "very active at one point. My partner is fine with this, but it isn't his thing. We're working through this."

On the other hand, some women won't put up with it at all, such as entrepreneur Rachel. "I don't like men who try to do their lord-high-super-dom nonsense on me," she sniffs. "I just laugh and walk away. They're silly."

Will You Share Her Wilder Side?

Yes, women have rich and varied fantasy lives, and many of them are willing to experiment with practices that were once considered taboo. In fact, we see the definition of "mainstream" sex becoming ever more fluid. So how important is it to women to find a partner who's willing to explore the outer limits with them?

The majority of women taking our survey feel it's somewhat important to find a partner who'll play along, but it isn't a make-or-break point. In fact, almost as many said it didn't make a difference to them. Their fantasies are *their* fantasies. "At the best," says entrepreneur Rachel, "we sort of fall into mutual fantasies together." Masters student Adrienne feels that "since my fantasies are more of the 'let's go have some great sex, just naked you and I' variety, it's not hard to find someone interested in the same."

A small percentage feels it's very important that their partners indulge them in their fantasies. As Sylvia, a 48-year-old marketing rep, puts it, "I try to accommodate what they enjoy, and I'd like fair play."

So be open to exploring her fantasies—especially if she's willing to explore yours. "Sometimes we'd like to play them out in the bedroom and want our partner to be willing to try it," says 27-year-old lawyer Blair. In the best of all possible worlds, her fantasies and yours will morph into something new and even more sizzling. As Roxie, a 25-year-old communications specialist, says about fantasies: "It's most fun to co-create them."

We couldn't agree more.

> **"I try to accommodate what they enjoy, and I'd like fair play."**
>
> **Sylvia, 48, marketing rep**

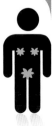

How important is it to you to find a partner willing to accommodate your fantasies?

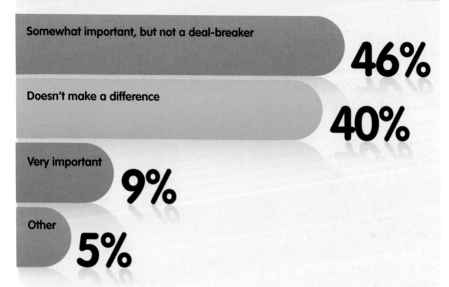

Somewhat important, but not a deal-breaker 46%

Doesn't make a difference 40%

Very important 9%

Other 5%

Note: Percentages may not equal 100% due to rounding.

How to Get a Woman *into* Bed: Secrets of Seduction

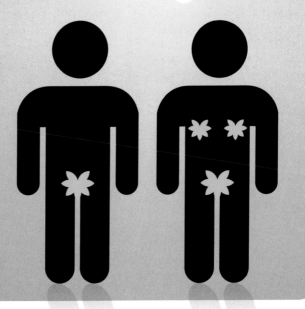

Thought you were finished? Not quite, boys! Knowing what to do *in* bed isn't going to help you very much if you can't get a woman *into* bed in the first place. And we're not talking about bar hookups, either. You could know her ten minutes or ten years; if you don't know what gets her hot for you, you're not going to get far.

Yes, we're talking about seduction.

Ah, sweet seduction. Whether you're married, dating, or single and working up the courage to ask someone out for the first time, seduction is one of the most important parts of a successful relationship, in and out of bed. Seduce her carefully and with forethought, and you've just paved the way not only to mind-blowing sex but also to a more rewarding relationship (if that's what you're both after). Seduce her badly or, worse yet, leave seduction out of the picture altogether, and you'll both feel dissatisfied and unappreciated . . . and the odds of you getting laid will drop dramatically.

Don't believe us? That's okay. We've come prepared with the opinions of three hundred other women, all of whom weighed in with their opinions and observations on what they wish men knew about the dance of seduction. These women will show you how to tell whether a woman is interested in going to bed with you in the first place, and if so, how to seduce her . . . or how to let her seduce you.

What Women Wish Men Knew about Seduction

Warning: Every woman is different. Yes, gentlemen, it's true. Although we all come with the same basic equipment, our needs and wants vary. This is a theme repeated throughout this book—and throughout life—so consider it a lesson worth taking to heart. It may save your life someday. Or at least lead to a more satisfying sex life for you and your partners.

In the words of Georgie, a 43-year-old editor, "We're all different, and are turned on (and off!) by different things. Don't assume that we'll like something just because another woman may have liked it. Be open-minded and pay attention to our response, and don't hesitate to ask what feels good or what we want if you're not sure. Always start off gently, unless you're told otherwise."

Twenty-nine-year-old Caroline, a teacher, puts it a little more emphatically: "You've GOT to ask us what we like and how we like it, or at least be willing to learn the body language that tells you what we want. You are NOT a perfect lover, even if you have been with some other woman. Every woman is different, and you have to let us know that you want to get it right and can take the hints." Or, as put quite simply by Jocelyn (who declined to give her age or profession, as many women did), "You don't know how to please every woman because you've pleased one."

So if a woman could tell you the *one* thing she wants you to know about seduction, what would she say? Sadly, there's no one universal truth that will get a woman into your bed every time, but there are some general themes. Here are a few insights into the female psyche when it comes to seduction.

Get to Know Her

Whether they're after a single night of hot sex or a long-term relationship, many women want to feel like a man is interested in them as a person, not just as a sex object. According to Andrea, a 40-year-old administrative manager, it's a definite aphrodisiac to "feel like he wants to get to know me in mind and body." And 35-year-old student Karen says, "Get to know me first. I'm turned on by your brain cells and clever wit. When we share common interests, activities, and values, I want to dive deeper. Discussing important issues and connecting emotionally opens me up to connecting on a physical level." Chloe agrees: "Sex is easier for me when there is a sense of familiarity. Getting to know what motivates someone, who he is, what he lives for, what his philosophies about life are, are all turn-ons."

Be aware, however, that sometimes a cigar is just a cigar. As Morgan, a 26-year-old graduate student, puts it, "Sometimes I just want you to listen to me. Me talking to you is not an invitation; more often than not, it's just that . . . me talking to you."

Show Her You Want Her. Scientists Say So.

"Focusing entirely on your partner is one of the sexiest things you can do," says Kelly. And she's not alone. Feeling like she's the center of your universe—at least for the time you're together—is a huge aphrodisiac for a lot of women. Holly says, "One of the sexiest things I have experienced is when the man makes it about pleasing me." Camilla, a 25-year-old advertising manager, agrees: "The most important thing to me is to feel wanted. If a guy is into my body and wants more of it, I get turned on." And Jyllian, a 44-year-old mom and engineer, says, "If you want to get a woman into bed, the best thing to do is actually be interested in her, what she says, what she does, what she thinks. In other words, the best way to a woman's crotch is through her brain."

Because for many women, like 27-year-old lawyer Blair, "It turns us on to see how much you want it and are into the idea of us seducing and initiating sex." Desire as an aphrodisiac. Who would have thunk it?

Well, scientists, for one. In a recent article, the *New York Times* reported that researchers are exploring the "critical part played by being desired" in a woman's libido. In the article, Marta Meana, a professor of psychology at the University of Nevada, Las Vegas, says that for women, "being desired is the orgasm." In other words, women want to know that you crave her beyond all control.

So don't phone it in, guys. Let a woman know you're interested in her mind and her body, and be there in the moment. Turn off the cell phone, shut down the laptop, and give the woman in front of you the same attention you would your favorite sports team. It'll be worth your while. As Mallory, a 26-year-old mother, sums it up, "Making a woman feel good about herself is the biggest turn-on." And if she's turned on, odds are you will be, too.

> **"If his look says I am the most beautiful woman in the world, then I am his."**
>
> **Elizabeth, 36, business owner**

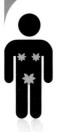

We Want You, Too . . . But Sometimes, It Takes Time

According to many of the women in our survey, men don't realize women are equally into them sexually—and not just for a relationship. Sometimes women just want good sex and don't want to feel badly about it. Sally, a 26-year-old coffee barista, says, "Not all women are looking for a husband or a relationship. Maybe they're just looking for good sex." Travel writer Shannon, 40, corroborates this: "Sometimes we just want sex." And 59-year-old clinical researcher Judy says, "We enjoy sex as much as you do! Talk nice, smell nice, and we'll go for it."

Even though we've established that women want and love sex, you can't rush them into it. Although women admit that they are as into sex as the men in their lives, they want to avoid the stigma of appearing "easy." Take it from Heather, a 25-year-old executive assistant, who says, "We really want to have sex right away, but often wait because we don't want to come off as a slut." This viewpoint is backed up by Rose, a 30-year-old teacher, who tells us, "We're constantly battling desire and guilt. We want to be with you, but we don't want to be perceived as easy. Men need to understand that and make us comfortable with that decision."

So let her set her own pace. Remember, patience is a virtue and sometimes virtue really is its own reward, at least according to Roxie, a 35-year-old communications professional: "Patience can be very sexy. If men honor my boundaries on the first couple of dates, don't make a fuss about it, and ask me out again, that's when I start looking

> **"If a man really wanted to have sex with me, I'd want him to be patient and have fun with me while waiting. He probably wouldn't have to wait that long."**
>
> **Annie, 62, writer**

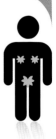

forward to the next date and hoping they'll be bolder in their moves." Although we'd never recommend playing games, "take your time and don't be pushy," says Annette. "Women know they can sleep with you or not." No one likes to be hounded or pressured. "While dating, don't try so hard," says Dawn, 42. "If it's gonna happen, it's gonna happen. Too much eagerness is annoying and boyish."

So let the object of your desire make up her mind in her own time and for her own reasons. "I've been on dates with men who thought they were seducing me but were in fact turning me off," says Annie. "They couldn't tell the difference. If a man really wanted to have sex with me, I'd want him to be patient and have fun with me while waiting. He probably wouldn't have to wait that long."

Gentlemen, Start Your Engines

Yet even when a woman lusts after you, she may still want you to make the first move. Sometimes it's as simple as wanting to know a man wants them. Says Troy, a 29-year-old lawyer, "I wish men didn't feel too vulnerable to make it obvious they want you. Being complimentary and eager is not a bad thing. Most women enjoy open desire." Paige (who didn't give us an age or profession) puts it this way: "I like it when men take initiative physically and emotionally. I don't like trying to guess whether someone likes me or not. I just wish they'd have the balls to say it."

So while women wait for their men to initiate, they try to send out signals giving their guys a green light. Unfortunately, men don't always read the signals—which can be frustrating to a woman who isn't comfortable making the first move. Defense attorney Lulu explains, "I wish men understood how hard it can be for us to initiate. If they don't respond positively, it can impact our willingness to initiate moving forward." And Bryn, a 41-year-old secretary, wishes men knew "how to read body language to understand when the woman is signaling it's okay to proceed to the next step. Nine years of marriage, and my husband still has no clue when I'm trying to drop him a hint that it's time to move in for the kill."

Casi has some advice on how you *can* tell she wants you: "If I'm kissing you passionately, if I am rubbing myself against you, if I seem unwilling to let the date end, chances are that I'm waiting for you to initiate." And project manager Pat, 56, backs this up with her own advice: "If a woman has taken the time to look and smell really nice (hair done, nails polished, legs shaved, new dress), if she's laughing at your jokes and touching you

lightly, go for it!" Or, as 22-year-old chemist Pearl puts it, "From my experience, women use skin to get men into bed."

Sometimes, though, the shoe is on the other foot. Women like Maren, a 33-year-old physical therapist, are waiting for a signal from you before reciprocating. "I tend to be a little slow on picking up on subtle clues," says Maren. "I need guys to let me know they're interested, without coming on too strong." Madison feels the same way. "If a man gives me some sort of signal to go ahead, I'll be very aggressive," she tells us. "But without the signal, I'll sit back and wait."

We thought Scarlet, a 34-year-old chef, summed it up perfectly. "Women try to be a little more subtle than men in letting someone know they're interested, but they often have to resort to being very obvious and blunt to get the message across," she

> **"If you're getting the vibe from a woman, let her know that you got it, so she doesn't have to beat you over the head with it!"**
>
> **Scarlet, 34, chef**

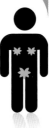

says. "If you're getting the vibe from a woman, let her know that you got it, so she doesn't have to beat you over the head with it!" Unless, of course, you like that sort of thing.

Let's Get Physical

Yeah, we know. It all seems very confusing and contradictory. But before you start hitting your head against a wall in frustration, we do have some practical advice as to what kind of signals women give to indicate their interest. Subtle touches are a good indicator that a woman is into you. She may not grab your package and say, "Do me now, big boy," but she *will* make contact. "If I touch you lightly," says Erika, a 50-year-old writer and teacher, "I'm interested." Adds Alicia, "The more times I 'accidentally' touch you, the more interested I am." Thirty-five-year-old teacher Taylor lets us in on this bit of insight: "Women flirt with their eyes, lightly touching a man's arm." Jennifer, a 34-year-old nonprofit worker, offers this advice: "If you're on a date and she's smiling and flirting and finding excuses to touch you, she wants you to kiss her. And probably a lot more!" Still don't get it? Liz, a 36-year-old physician, puts it very bluntly: "If a woman touches you, she wants you."

However (oh, come on, you didn't think it would be *that* simple, did you?), an important distinction here is whether a woman's interest means she's willing to go the distance that particular day or night. Sometimes it's just the first step. According to 66-year-old writer Marisol, "Affection is a prelude to closeness, which is a prelude to sex." Cautions Caroline, a 29-year-old teacher, "If I'm touching you during our conversation, it probably means I'm interested, but it's not necessarily a green light for THAT NIGHT . . . especially if we've just met."

So don't rush it. Unless she wants you to. And the best way to figure *that* out is to learn how to read those signals, be they flirtatious banter, more direct statements ("Take me now, baby!"), or more subtle physical nuances, such as the brush of her hand on your arm or thigh, or a steamy kiss while she grinds her body against yours. You can also pay attention to our next tip.

Approach Her with Subtlety

Let's talk about subtlety, those little nuances in the courtship dance that can make the difference between a romantic pas de deux and a clumsy faux pas. "Don't try so hard," cautions Gayle, a 38-year-old writer. "Sometimes it's all about subtlety." And 32-year-old business executive Suzy says, "Subtlety and patience work best. Make her *want* it and long for it way before you make your move. That could be several dates after you think it may be."

Monica, a 49-year-old restaurant owner, says you'd be well advised to "plant subtle seeds of sexual desire in your conversation and touch that will pique her desire." Although some women like the Neanderthal approach, "gentle persuasion and intelligence work better than brute force and ignorance," says Nara, a 41-year-old massage therapist. Grape agrees. "I wish men knew that a few neck nibbles, lingering glances, and adoration will go way further in seduction than the caveman 'me like you' approach," she says. It will also help her relax, letting both of you enjoy each other's company. "When a man is less physically aggressive, it allows the woman to feel safe and allow playfulness to unwind and flow," says Embe, a 52-year-old bodyworker.

Pay Close Attention

It's not all about *you* practicing subtlety, however. Your partner's signals might be quite subtle themselves, which is why you need to pay close attention. Thirty-three-year-old marketing professional Stacey reminds that "sex is an ongoing process. If we want to have sex, we throw signs out there all the time." Refer back to the tip about those light touches. . . . Heather, a 37-year-old dolphin trainer, puts it simply: "When we're standing there closing our eyes with our heads tilted up at you, you're supposed to kiss us." If you can't trust a dolphin trainer to give you signals, then who can you trust? At least she's not asking you to jump through hoops.

Keep It Real

No game players need apply. The message from our survey respondents is clear: Be yourself. Twenty-nine-year-old public relations executive Dawn had this to say: "Take the hint! If I want you, and you want me, reciprocate. No games." Kate, a 34-year-old physician, agrees. "I like men to be direct," Kate says. "I hate playing games and trying to guess what men are thinking."

Honesty is definitely the best policy, at least according to the following women:

> "Honesty is very sexy; lying and hustling are not."
> **Francesca, 39, education professional**

> "Seduction isn't about saying what you *think* a woman wants to hear. It's way sexier when a guy is direct and honest about what he wants."
> **Hope, age and occupation withheld**

> "Being super suave and smooth is not attractive. It's like you've done it a million times. Being nervous or not smooth is endearing, and makes me feel special."
> **Sara, 27, CPA**

"Be genuinely into the woman. She can tell when you are. Ask good questions, listen, be yourself."

Carrie, 38, entrepreneur

And don't feel like you have to make a big production out of it all, either. "It's the little things that count," advises 33-year-old graduate student Adrienne. "Show your interest and be sincere." And how do you show your interest? "Come up and talk to me like I'm one of the boys," says Elizabeth. "Be at ease and make it clear to me you're interested." And although not all women want to talk about beer and football, they *are* interested in communication as a prelude to sex. Thirty-two-year-old Alli tells us, "Just being nice and talking is the best way to seduce a girl."

You didn't know it was so easy, did you?

A Little Romance Goes a Long Way

That fantasy of wanting Prince Charming to come riding in on a white stallion as the answer to all our problems? For the majority of women, it's pretty much a thing of the past. The desire for romance, however, is as strong as ever. Flowers, candlelight, chocolate, sweet passionate kisses . . . it's all good. Cari, a 26-year-old administrative assistant, tells us, "We like to be seduced. We are all for 'it,' but want to feel as if you're making an effort to make it romantic!"

Most women don't expect diamonds or $200 bottles of champagne, either. Destiny says, "It isn't that complicated or expensive. Just pay her compliments, and be yourself. Pick a flower in the park on the way to your date, and you've already won multiple bonus points!" It's all about the little gestures that tell a woman you find her beautiful and desirable. Try "romantic gestures—e.g., little scribbled notes, messages on the mirror," says Arianna, a 33-year-old household engineer. "The little things count big!"

Try to avoid being too goal-oriented— a hard thing to do nowadays. Kayla tells us, "Seduction for women is more of an overall sensual experience." In other words, there's more to it than putting a quarter in the slot and getting a quick ride. For instance, many women listed the art of kissing as high on their list of how to seduce them successfully. "Kissing is very important," affirms 50-year-old artist Jackie. "Don't skimp on the kissing, and try to be really good at it." January, a 45-year-old paralegal, simply states, "Kissing is seductive."

And remember to have fun! Says Michelle, a 35-year-old marketing manager, "When we're seducing a man, it's not in hopes of getting jumped within ten minutes. We want to enjoy the game of flirtation with someone who knows it's going to lead to bed eventually, but not for a while. Enjoy the dance. *Play!*"

Use Your Brains!

Are you ready for the most important glimpse into the female psyche you'll ever get? Here it is. "The biggest sexual organ is the brain," says Sylvia, a 38-year-old marketing rep. "If you can't turn that on, the rest is unimportant."

If you want to seduce a woman, start with her mind and her imagination. Men are visual creatures and easily turned on; for most women, it's a little more involved. Remember Cyrano de Bergerac, the famous hotheaded swordsman and eloquent wordsmith who (anonymously) seduced the love of his life via his words and letters? Women are creatures of the mind and imagination, and intellectual foreplay generally occurs before any actual touching has occurred. "Engage my mind and my imagination first," says Jackie. "Seduce me with words, be they written or verbal, and you'll already have a head start with the foreplay." Forty-six-year-old writer Inara agrees, adding, "And keep the seduction sensual as opposed to sexual." And Alina, a 25-year-old academic bum, says this about her dates: "Intellectual stimulation plays a huge part in whether or not they'll score."

So how would we sum up these responses, opinions, and bits of advice on the art of seduction? Yes, they varied widely, but we think that the critical ingredient is self-confidence. "Women are attracted to confidence," says Sunny, a 36-year-old project manager. "This is different from aggression, which results from either insecurity or horniness, both of which can be turnoffs." Be direct about your interest, without being pushy. We think Shelley, a 38-year-old artist, says it best: "Courting is seductive. A hard sell is awful."

"The biggest sexual organ is the brain. If you can't turn that on, the rest is unimportant."

Sylvia, 38, marketing rep

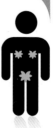

What's the First Thing Women Notice about a Guy?

Okay, before we discuss such important topics as who should make the first move, what's guaranteed to send a woman running for the exit, and whether it's the size of your bank account or the size of your manly package that's more important, let's start with the basics: What's the first thing a woman notices about you at that all-so-important initial meeting? Although first impressions don't always make or break a potential pairing, they *are* important.

Appearance matters, but …

A whopping 70 percent of women surveyed admitted that a man's appearance definitely tops the list of what she notices first. As Chloe says, "The first thing has to be physical appearance. It's impossible not to see someone when you first notice them."

Let's face it. Our society places a high value on beauty. And thanks to years of indoctrination in Hollywood's airbrushed standards of appearance, many people are sometimes led to expect unrealistically high standards in themselves and their partners. And even if a woman doesn't expect you to live up to the six-pack-abs eye candy abounding in movies

What is the first thing you notice about a guy?

Physical appearance **70%**

Personality **19%**

Other **10%**

2% Economic status

1% The size of his package proudly bulging in his pants

Note: *Percentages may not equal 100% due to rounding.*

Think about what you find attractive in a guy's appearance. How important are each of the following physical attributes to you?

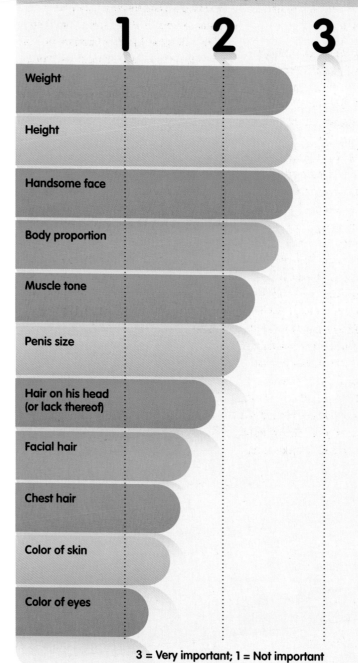

	1	**2**	**3**
Weight			
Height			
Handsome face			
Body proportion			
Muscle tone			
Penis size			
Hair on his head (or lack thereof)			
Facial hair			
Chest hair			
Color of skin			
Color of eyes			

3 = Very important; 1 = Not important

like *300*, she's still most likely to check out your butt before your personality the first time she sees you. But before you start feeling discouraged, read on.

For you fellows who don't look like movie stars or even reality TV stud muffins, don't despair. Because even though appearance topped the charts in percentage, most women included a caveat: Yes, they notice a man's appearance first, but without something else to back it up, good looks only go so far. "I selected personality first," says Hailey (who was also shy about sharing her age and career path), "but then had to select physical appearance because it HAS to be the 'first' thing one notices. But it may not be among the most important 'first things.'" Forty-seven-year-old marketing rep Sylvia agrees. "Great looks will catch my eye, just as a beautiful anything does. What draws my eyes back is an air about them. The way they laugh or hold their head. I've been attracted to men not classically handsome, but the inner personality makes them attractive." Beth, a 43-year-old designer, also admits that although good looks are what initially attract her, "sparkly wit, intelligence, mischief keep me in the game. They can also make up for plain looks."

Even after an initial positive first reaction to a man's hunky appearance, it's clear that good looks alone are not enough. For instance, Roxie, a 35-year-old communications professional, is more interested in what she calls his "tricks and his manners." Roxie adds, "Obviously, striking looks (one way or the other) will always catch my attention, but what keeps me NOTICING is a man's way of interacting with people—and particularly women, though not just me."

"I notice appearance first," agrees Rachel, a 45-year-old entrepreneur, "but that doesn't hold my attention if he opens his mouth and is stupid, mean, or boring." And Jennifer, a 31-year-old nonprofit worker, makes this distinction: "If you really mean 'notice,' then it's physical appearance because it's the first thing I see. BUT if you really mean what first attracts me to a guy, it's personality (with appearance a close second)."

So yes, though an initially pleasing physical package will catch a woman's eye, it won't keep her attention without substance behind it.

It's All About Personality

Some women don't care what a guy looks like. If he has a lousy personality, it doesn't matter if he's a cross between Brad Pitt, Clive Owen, and Daniel Craig (with a little Hugh Jackman tossed in for that Wolverine appeal); he still won't be getting any, at least not from Monica, a 49-year-old restaurant owner. "Confidence and personality," says Monica, "can override the importance of exterior looks in any of the categories." Karen, a 35-year-old student, agrees: "If his personality is lacking, I'm not getting physical!" And just in case there are any lingering doubts, Judy, a 59-year-old clinical researcher, states unequivocally, "Personality will always super-sede any physical traits.

Make Me Laugh!

Interestingly enough, even though our survey results showed percentages in favor of physical appearance, our respondents' additional comments leaned heavily toward personality over good looks. For instance, according to several women ranging from their 20s to late 50s, a good sense of humor and a ready smile are at least as important as a well-chiseled jaw and good pecs.

Roxie, our 35-year-old communications expert, had this to say about personality: "I notice when men are playful, lighthearted, and ready to smile or laugh. It's the subtleties that keep me rapt." Summer, a 27-year-old TV advertising exec, said, "Certain elements, like personality and sense of humor, automatically make many of these physical attributes less weighted. If a man had a sparkling personality and made me laugh, then I'd be willing to sacrifice some of the physical attributes that are normally deal-breakers."

Further backing up this opinion is Annette, a 44-year-old in middle management, who says, "Appearance doesn't matter that much. Personality, intelligence, and a clever sense of humor are most important." "I find a good sense of humor MUCH sexier than a full head of hair," says 43-year-old artist and writer Julie, "but if he has no hair, he'd better compensate for it with a good sense of humor!"

Our conclusion: For sexual efficacy, a sense of humor is cheaper and easier than investing in Rogaine or Hair Club for Men, gents!

Be Smart About It!

Although some women may be content with the male equivalent of eye candy, not all are satisfied with a guy just because he's "really, really, really good-looking" (to quote *Zoolander*). Nearly 79 percent of our respondents rated intelligence as the most important trait in a man (closely followed by a good sense of humor, good hygiene, emotional stability, and maturity). In other words, pheromones may arouse initial interest, but a lot of women need mental stimulation to take the next step. "Frankly," says 35-year-old college professor Alex, "if he's cute but not smart, I'm turned off in about five minutes. Where's the bubble [checkbox] for 'brain'?" Annie, a 62-year-old writer, concurs with Alex: "I'm interested in what lies behind the looks: i.e., the brain."

Dress for Success

Dressing well was only at the top of the charts for 8 percent of the women taking our survey, but style does weigh in to some degree in terms of how some women perceive your attractiveness. Carrie, a 28-year-old entrepreneur, admits, "I often associate good looks with economic status. Nice dresser, good body, probably has money to support that." Forty-five-year-old Rachel, another entrepreneur, has a slightly less mercenary take on it, saying, "Sometimes good style can overcome average looks."

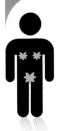

"I notice appearance first, but that doesn't hold my attention if he opens his mouth and is stupid, mean, or boring."

Rachel, 45, entrepreneur

What Part of Your Body Does She Find the Sexiest?

We also asked women to rate their favorite body parts on a man. You know, if they were playing Dr. Victoria Frankenstein, which parts would they be the pickiest about stealing from the graveyard or morgue?

Our survey results showed that our potential female Frankensteins would take the most care picking out eyes and shoulders, tied at 21 percent each, for their manly monsters. From the women for whom the eyes have it: Annie, a 62-year-old writer, says, "I have fallen in love with men of many shapes and sizes (although generally slender and medium height prevail), but always with beautiful or at least expressive eyes." Pat, a 56-year-old project manager, had this to say: "Dark expressive eyes. Honestly, with my current husband, I fell in love with the wrinkles around the corners of his eyes. They ray out like sunbeams, indicating a man who spends a lot of time in the sun, and a man who smiles much. They truly are 'laugh lines.'"

Ladies who voted shoulders as their particular favorite part of the male anatomy were more to the point: Ulla, a 27-year-old performer, says, "I love a man with a strong back and broad shoulders," whereas Beth, a 43-year-old designer, puts it this way: "A man with skinny shoulders is a turnoff."

Legs and butt also have their fans among the ladies. "LOVE a good pair of gams on a guy," says Inara, a 46-year-old writer. "None of that skinny rock-star pipe-stem crap." Her fondness for well-muscled legs is shared by Jackie (another survey participant who wants to keep her age and profession a secret). "I love good legs on a guy," she says. "Muscle tone, not skinny rock-star legs. If a guy has good Toshiro Mifune–type thighs, it makes up for lack of tone in other places." (Note: Guys, if you don't know who Toshiro Mifune is, rent the movie *Seven Samurai*. It'll either inspire sessions with the leg press machine at the gym or some kendo lessons. Either way, you'll get great thighs!)

And because you need something to connect those gorgeous legs to the rest of the body, 40-year-old admin manager Andrea is especially fond of the male derriere: "It's not just about the shape and size of their ass but even more importantly how they carry their ass. Something about the energy in their walk or something. It's hard to explain." That's okay, Andrea. We'll just call it the je ne sais quoi of masculine buttocks and leave it at that.

There were even a couple of fans of hips and hip bones:

"The hip bones in particular."
Rose, 30, teacher

"I love firm pecs, but collarbones and hip bones are a close second."
Karen, 35, student

What male body part do you find the absolute sexiest?

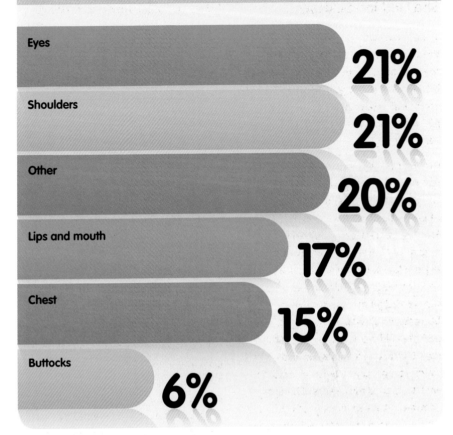

Eyes **21%**

Shoulders **21%**

Other **20%**

Lips and mouth **17%**

Chest **15%**

Buttocks **6%**

Note: *Percentages may not equal 100% due to rounding.*

"More specifically, the 'V thing' formed by the hip bones, waist, and pelvic area."
Lula, 30, librarian

And in case your best feature hasn't been mentioned yet, here are some other popular traits:

"Voice."
Kary, age and profession withheld (We're assuming she's talking about a man's tone as opposed to just having working vocal chords.)

"Teeth!!! Good teeth!!!"
Yvette, age and profession withheld (We suspect Yvette is a carnivore.)

"Nice tall V shape."
Nana, 37, marketing manager

"Broad, muscular or chunky, clean, hairless."
Shai, 33, marketer (Vin Diesel wannabes, are you reading this?)

"For me, it's weight. I just like a skinny, gangly guy."
Emily, 30, attorney (Napoleon Dynamites of the world, pay attention!)

"I do like luscious hair and lips!"
Beth, 43, designer

"The triangular indentation that cyclists get just above the knee can be amazingly sexy."
Ginger, 38, project manager

Just goes to show there really is something for everyone.

Then there's the matter of body hair. Pat, a 56-year-old project manager, likes it, telling us, "I'm drawn to a certain 'type,' which includes a hairy chest." Yet Ellen, a 37-year-old Web development team manager, disagrees: "I find too much chest hair a turnoff." So does 43-year-old designer Beth, who put it this way: "Furry guys are a turnoff."

Facial hair also got a general thumbs-down. "Facial hair," says Karren, a 45-year-old attorney, "is only important because I don't like it." And if you've got a beard, you won't be kissing 30-year-old entrepreneur Carrie: "Facial hair, to me, is gross. Think of that scraping against my baby face? No, thanks."

A few women mentioned that height was an issue for them. "I'm very tall," says Sara, a 27-year-old CPA, "so height in a guy is very important to me. It's my only make-or-break." Twenty-eight-year-old medical office manager Jenny concurs. "I'm 5'8," Jenny states, "so I want them to be taller than me."

By the way, ears didn't get any votes, so anyone out there with Spock-like ears or the proverbial jug handles can breathe easier. Evidently, no one is looking.

Hands Down!

To our embarrassment, we forgot to list a body part that was very popular among our survey respondents: hands. Considering the part hands play in foreplay, we weren't surprised at the following comment from Troy, a 26-year-old lawyer: "Hands, hands, hands! You missed the most exciting physical attributes: hands and smile. I know lots of women have a thing about hands. If you are a long-fingered man, you don't want to know the things I'm thinking about you." (Um . . . Troy, we suspect they DO want to know what you're thinking about them.) Bryn, a 41-year-old secretary, had this to say: "The number-one thing I look for in a man's appearance are his HANDS. That's the first thing I look at, before I waste time deciding whether the rest of his body is attractive. Shape, size, and grooming are all very important when it comes to his hands." And 34-year-old Jennifer, who works in the nonprofit sector, says, "I love men's hands. Maybe because I want them on me. Who knows?"

And just in case you still have any doubts:

> "I always notice men's hands."
> **Jane, 39, businesswoman**

> "Hands would actually be my first choice."
> **Mallory, 26, mother**

> "Well-formed, intelligent, and clean hands are incredibly sexy."
> **Melanie, 25, graduate student**

So clean under those fingernails, boys.

It All Depends . . .

But wait a second. Says Annabelle: "It depends 100 percent on the guy." Like Annabelle, many women, even after stating definite preferences for specific body parts and types, are willing to toss everything out the window if the right guy comes along. "Each guy is different," 26-year-old graduate student Morgan tells us. "So naturally, each guy has his own sexiest body part." Inara, a 46-year-old writer, says, "A lot of what's attractive to me depends on how it's all put together on a guy and whether or not I find his personality attractive." (There's that pesky personality issue again!) Pat, a 56-year-old project manager, adds, "It matters more to me that a man is comfortable in his own body, whatever that shape may be, than whether that body type appeals to me."

And according to Helena, a 39-year-old professor, it's often a matter of proportionality, "especially in terms of how a man 'fits' your own body." But sometimes "it really depends on what's in front of me at the time," says Julie, a 43-year-old writer and artist, "and what he's doing with what he's got!"

Totally confused now? Don't be. We encourage you guys to think of it as an opportunity to make the most out of what you have, rather than worry about what you're lacking. Go forth with confidence. Because as Ginger, a 38-year-old project manager, sums it up: "Insecurity is never attractive."

The Brass Tacks of Seduction

So you see a woman who catches your eye. What's your next move to signal your interest and let her know you'd like to get her know her better? The ladies were pretty straightforward when answering this question. Flirting and playfulness topped the list at 29 percent, with eye contact a fairly close second at 19 percent. A direct smile, light touches, and showing an interest in her ran neck-in-neck for third place.

Thirty-nine-year-old professor Helena goes for guys who know how to combine techniques. "Eye contact, then a smile," says Helena, "and asking questions to demonstrate interest in me." Holly prefers a more direct approach: "Tell me he's interested in me. Blunt communication works, because I don't have to guess."

Flirting, by the way, does not mean whipping out tired old lines of the "Hey, baby, what's *your* sign?" variety, nor does it mean slapping her on the butt or groping her (although 1 percent of our survey respondents indicated groping is an appropriate way to show your interest) after a drink or two. Flirting is the art of making another person feel interesting and attractive, which includes listening to her and paying attention to her mood. Combine that with some well-placed and subtle light touches on the arm, hand, or small of the back, and you'll take the ambiguity out of the whole "does he or doesn't he?" phase of the courtship game.

> **"Tell me he's interested in me. Blunt communication works, because I don't have to guess."**
>
> **Holly**

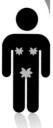

If you find a man attractive, how important to you are each of the following personality life traits?

Trait	1	2	3	4

- Intelligence
- Good sense of humor
- Good hygiene
- Emotional stability
- Maturity
- Self-confidence
- Good social skills
- Ability to commit
- Ability to give you an orgasm
- Education
- Good social network
- Well-dressed
- Income
- Similar political view
- Occupation
- Similar religion

4 = Very important; 1 = Not important

Game Killers

So you're past that first nerve-wracking hurdle of whether or not she's interested in you. She's definitely intrigued. So how do you take it to the next level? How about we tell you what *not* to do if you're serious about a second date, let alone getting her into bed?

And we have a winner, folks, with rudeness to your date or others garnering nearly a fourth of the votes for behavior most likely to send a woman running for the door. According to project manager Pat, 56, "ogling other women, or making me feel like he's got me as his 'backup plan' in case nothing better comes along" definitely qualifies as rude. Heather, a 31-year-old song artist, says a surefire way to kill the deal with her is someone who "disrespects me or others around me."

So remember, if you treat the waitstaff at a restaurant with disrespect or pay too much attention to your waitress's cleavage, odds are your date will be thinking of a way to cut things short before the dessert course.

Self-absorbed and selfish behavior didn't rate too much lower on the "things that irritate me" list. Guys who are more interested in their own appearance than that of their date don't win points with 36-year-old swim instructor Frankie, whose least favorite trait in a date is someone who "talks about his physique. That's the worst." And says Hailey,

"A too-well-dressed guy is kind of a turnoff. I'm not interested in someone who is terribly fussy about his appearance."

Physical aggressiveness and lousy hygiene were right behind Narcissus and his mirror. In fact, Esra lumps them all together as equally irritating and says, "I'd rank a bunch of these equally: poor hygiene, self-absorbed, rude, too aggressive."

Ginger, however, couldn't pick just one. "So many of these apply I can't pick one to be the worst." She wasn't the only woman to feel this way. As 35-year-old defense attorney Lulu puts it, "How am I supposed to choose just one of these? These all suck."

Talking too much and making bad, off-color jokes were two of the least offensive traits, only getting 0.5 percent and 1.5 percent respectively. Insisting on paying for things didn't get any votes at all (no big surprise), although one of our respondents, Turner, stated bluntly, "Nice men = boring." Which means there might be hope for you BlackBerry-addicted, self-absorbed fellows after all.

And even if you get through an entire date without stepping into any of these potentially nasty piles of behavioral crap, it's still possible to screw it up in the last five minutes by getting too cocky. This from 36-year-old business owner Elizabeth: "I once had a guy close off the date after a goodnight kiss by asking me, 'So, are you wet now?' Why would ANY man think that is appropriate?!" Why indeed.

How Soon Is Too Soon (or Not Soon Enough)?

So you made it past the first date, maybe even a second and third as well. How soon can you expect a woman to go to bed with you once it's been established she's attracted to you?

The answers varied widely on this one. For instance, Jane, our 39-year-old business-woman, is basically of the "it's now or never" mind-set. "If I haven't had sex with someone within the first three dates," she says, "I don't ever want to have sex with him." Mae, a 30-year-old graduate student, agrees, saying she usually sleeps with a man "after our first date, though it depends also on other factors."

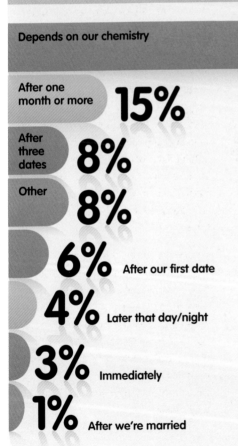

How quickly do you want to have sex after meeting a man who attracts you?

- Depends on our chemistry — **55%**
- After one month or more — **15%**
- After three dates — **8%**
- Other — **8%**
- **6%** After our first date
- **4%** Later that day/night
- **3%** Immediately
- **1%** After we're married

Note: *Percentages may not equal 100% due to rounding.*

Other women have a three-date minimum even if they're interested in the guy right off the bat. Although she's now married, swim instructor Frankie tells us that in her single days, "Sometimes I would want to have sex immediately, but I would wait until after the third date." And Carrie, a 40-year-old scientist, says, "I may want to have sex later that day, but I try to wait till after a few dates."

Why do women want to wait? Some want to get to know the guy better; others see it as a reputation issue. Dawn, a 42-year-old domestic executive, puts it this way: "This is the answer I'll tell my kid: at least three dates."

Other women are even more cautious. For instance, 20-year-old student Kyleranne will not sleep with someone until "after we have established feelings for each other and I know the relationship is going somewhere." And Heather, our photographer, usually waits "about a month or more . . . but it also depends."

What it depends *on* is that elusive quality known as chemistry. Sometimes physical compatibility can grow over time as couples become comfortable with one another and discover hidden qualities in each other. But 55 percent of the women we surveyed said the amount of time they take before sleeping with someone depends on chemistry. According to 48-year-old Sylvia, a marketing rep, "I might *know* I'd enjoy sex, but it depends on chemistry and other factors as to whether I act on it."

And because we always have a wild card or two in the deck, we'll share what 35-year-old writer Kate had to say: "There's a difference between when you *want* to and when you *will*." Carrie, the entrepreneur, confirms this: "I *want* to wait one month or more, but oftentimes I don't have that kind of restraint and it winds up being more like a few dates."

In other words, a woman may have some very definite ideas about when she wants to go to bed with you, but you never know what might just change her mind. Good luck, gentlemen.

You Go First.
No, YOU Go First!

Whether you're in a relationship or single, who suggests getting busy? Do you come up with some dazzling one-liner guaranteed to sweep her off her feet or wait for her to make the first move? We asked women how often they like to take the initiative and got these results: "Sometimes" is the winner at a whopping 58 percent, followed by the ubiquitous "it depends on the man and the situation" at 20 percent. Not very helpful, we know. But unfortunately (or fortunately), there aren't any hard-and-fast rules that apply to all women. Let's see if we can clarify this a bit.

Approach #1: Let's Split It Down the Middle

Many women are happy either being the initiator or the initiatee, as long as they get equal time in both roles. It prevents either partner from feeling the onus of always having to be the supplicant when they want to have sex. Vanessa, a 35-year-old administrator, has this complaint: "In my marriage, it ends up being me taking the lead 90 percent of the time. I'd like to have to only 40 to 50 percent of the time." Seems fair. And Vanessa isn't the only woman who feels this way.

"It should go both ways and both should be comfortable with that," says Annette, a 42-year-old manager. "I'd say 50/50 on this one," agrees Adrienne, a 33-year-old graduate student. "Sometimes I want to be in charge, and sometimes I want to be tossed around." Ginger, a 38-year-old project manager, puts it in slightly more elemental terms: "I like to switch off between the prey and predator roles."

> **"I like to switch off between the prey and predator roles."**
>
> **Ginger, 38, project manager**

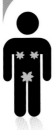

Approach #2: Come and Get Me, Big Boy

Some women definitely favor the old-fashioned approach. That is to say, they prefer to be approached rather than take the initiative. "It's true," 35-year-old communications professional Roxie tells us. "I'm an old-fashioned girl and RARELY make the first move. Part of the turn-on for me is being pursued, and having the man initiate is key in the art of seduction." Matilda, a 32-year-old pharmacist, says, "I like to be seduced. I need to feel like he's the boss." Christina, a 32-year-old in marketing, doesn't "have a problem seducing a man, but it's always preferable to be pursued."

Several of our respondents said they just weren't comfortable making the first move. "I can send signals," says Seraphin, a 40-year-old technology strategist, "but I sort of feel like a ho if I take the initiative." Says Casi, "As in dancing, I prefer the man to lead."

And then there's the issue of practicality brought up by 33-year-old Stacey, a marketing professional: "I'm a mother of a two-year-old. Rarely am I the initiator. I'm just too damn tired!"

That's definitely something to keep in mind, gentlemen, if you're a parent or involved with the mother of an infant or toddler. She may need that extra inspiration brought on by your show of interest. Just be sensitive to the timing! "Don't try to initiate anything—let alone sex—when I'm changing a diaper or dealing with a full-on tantrum," says Roxanne, a 45-year-old writer and mother of a preschooler. Of course, any guy who thinks sexy thoughts during either occasion might need therapy, but that's another topic for another book.

> ## "Sometimes I want to be in charge, and sometimes I want to be tossed around."
>
> **Adrienne, 33, graduate student**

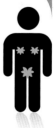

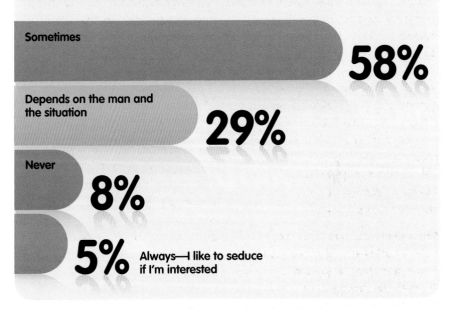

Whether you're in a relationship or single, how often do you like to take the sexual initiative?

Sometimes — **58%**

Depends on the man and the situation — **29%**

Never — **8%**

5% Always—I like to seduce if I'm interested

Note: *Percentages may not equal 100% due to rounding.*

Approach #3: Did We Mention It All Depends?

Some women are mellow about the subject, willing to go with the flow. "When I'm in a relationship," says 46-year-old writer Inara, "I've rarely had to take the initiative, but I like to do so once in a while to keep things interesting and fresh." And Bryn, a 41-year-old secretary, declares, "Typically, I like being 'ravished,' but with a guy who's hesitant, I don't mind taking the lead." For Heather, a 28-year-old travel photographer, it all depends on the stage of the relationship: "He can initiate at first, but after we're comfortable, then I do sometimes."

But even women who are in long-term relationships don't always want to be in the role of lingerie-clad seductress, tugging on their partner's sleeves while begging, "Honey, I got a real need for some lovin'!" It can actually take a toll on a woman's self-esteem and libido to always have to be the one expressing interest first. As 56-year-old Pat puts it, "I'm in a very-long-term marriage. Unfortunately, I usually end up taking the initiative, but I'd rather it not always be me."

According to Jennifer, a 34-year-old who works in the nonprofit sector, switching roles with your partner can be a real turn-on.

"I often find myself taking the sexual initiative (which is fine), so I do find it very sexy when it's the man who takes the lead." And even those women who don't mind initiating just don't want to have to do it all the time. "Partners aren't mind readers," says Frankie. "I'm married, and I'm more than happy to do the initiating when I want it. But I wouldn't like it if I had to do it all of the time. It is really give-and-take."

If you're looking for a relationship, it's not always a good thing when a woman takes the initiative, as illustrated by 24-year-old scientist Paris. "If I'm trying to seduce you after we've just met, it's probably because I'm looking to get laid," she says, "not because you're any more special than any other guy around that night." And Roxanne, a 45-year-old writer, states that "just because we want to sleep with you fairly early on in the relationship, it doesn't mean we're sluts, nor does it mean we want a relationship with you. Maybe we're just attracted to you and like sex. Don't hold it against us."

> "Typically, I like being 'ravished,' but with a guy who's hesitant, I don't mind taking the lead."
>
> Bryn, 41, secretary

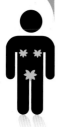

How to Keep Things Going

So you've connected with a woman, possibly gone to bed with her, and you'd like things to continue. To this end, we asked women what personality or life traits are important to them once they find a man attractive. In other words, what seals the deal? Top of the list, as we discussed earlier in the chapter, were intelligence and a sense of humor. Here are some others.

Emotional Stability Equals Sexy

We could have also titled this tip "Nice guys finish first," because emotional stability came next on the list along with traits like maturity, self-confidence, and good social skills. Most mentally healthy women want a man who has his act together. "I've learned that this trait is very important after dating men who were *not* emotionally stable!" says Sunny, a 36-year-old project manager. It also seems some women aren't as interested in sexual prowess as they are in finding a man who is basically a good guy. "If he is emotionally unstable, he'll never get close enough for me to find out whether or not he can give me an orgasm," says Pat, 56, a project manager.

Despite what you may think or see in the media, not all women are looking for the proverbial "bad boy," because, as sexy as a player can be in theory, he's not exactly what a gal wants in a long-term relationship. And women aren't just looking for a man who nice to *them*—they want someone who cares for others in general, even strangers.

Thirty-two-year-old Elizabeth, a mental health provider, is definitely looking for a man who is "kind to my family and friends." And for entrepreneur Rachel, "Compassion is absolutely essential."

Become a Giver—of Orgasms

How important is a man's ability—or even willingness—to help a woman achieve orgasm during sex? Very (although it actually came after "ability to commit" among our respondents). According to 44-year-old Annette, "I've been with men who felt that my orgasm was optional. It is not."

Some women, though still looking for the Big O, have a slightly different view of the situation. Marla, a 30-year-old artist, discovered that patience was the answer. "I almost broke up with my now-husband because it took almost a month for me to orgasm when we were first together," she says. "We got over that hump quickly." Forty-five-year-old attorney Karren doesn't mind being patient, either. "The ability to give me an orgasm doesn't matter at the beginning because I figure I can teach him that," she says. "But if he still doesn't get it after a while, then it becomes important."

Some women noted that an inability to climax with a partner has more to do with the woman than the man. Roxie, our communications professional, says, "I've never *not* been able to have an orgasm with a partner.

I think that has more to do with *me* than my partner, so if I can't communicate to him what I want and like, he's definitely not the right guy for me—I'm holding back for a reason." Also advocating personal responsibility is Shai, a 33-year-old marketer. "One myth about women is that it's the *man* who can't give us an orgasm. It's us not letting them. We need to let go and help them help us—and get ourselves in the mood, too."

Many women just want to know their man is trying to do their best. Says Seraphin, a 40-year-old technology strategist, "The show *Sex and the City* (Samantha and her trials in particular) make me try to appreciate a guy more, even though he may have a smaller-than-desired body part or not give me great orgasms in the beginning. As long as he TRIES to do better, then nature finds a way." And who says television doesn't contribute something positive to society?

Elizabeth, a 36-year-old business owner, sums it up this way: "If I don't have an orgasm, I don't blame them. To me, it's more important that they act like they want to be with ME and that I'm the most beautiful person in the world to them. That's orgasmic."

The Miscellaneous Factor

And just in case you were getting complacent and thinking you knew what works, we have to once again remind you that ever woman is different. Some women want a guy who can love *and* talk: "I've found when the sex and the conversation really work, a relationship can go anywhere," says writer Annie, 62. Forty-three-year-old Beth has a longer list. "He needs to be passionate about what he does," she says. "And have fun. And know how to take care of himself and others. And love animals." At least she didn't ask for a cure for cancer!

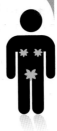

"I've found when the sex and the conversation really work, a relationship can go anywhere."

Annie, 62, writer

Acknowledgments

First and foremost, thanks to Dave Fitzgerald, whose enthusiasm and assistance (not to mention his willingness to assist in hands-on research) were essential to the writing of this book.

And let me not forget Cynthia's husband, Nima, whose sense of humor brought fun—and beautiful charts—to the project!

Gratitude to all the survey respondents and their willingness to share their thoughts and desires. I know so much more about many of my friends than I ever thought possible . . .

Kudos to Jill and Quiver for letting me join Cynthia on this project, Tere for her editing skills and friendly, diplomatic personality, and Sheree B. for handling all those pesky legal details!

And last and foremost (can I do that?), thanks and affection to my coauthor and friend, without whom I would never have expanded my writing repertoire to erotica, both nonfiction and fiction, and whose patience, enthusiasm, and talent made her an absolute joy to work with!

—**Dana Fredsti**

I hate writing acknowledgments. They never completely express what I want them to say as eloquently as I'd like to say it. For example, how do I begin to thank my husband, Nima, who very simply made it possible for me to embark on this project by taking care of our son so I could sneak off to write? That's only a tiny example of the support he gave me, and has given me, with every project. (And, as Dana mentions, there are the beautiful charts.)

Nor can I begin to thank Dave Fitzgerald enough. He's been with us every step of the way, with good humor and cheerfulness.

Like Dana, I have to also thank our survey respondents for being so willing to open up to us with such amazing candor.

I also want to thank our agent, Sheree Bykofsky of Sheree Bykofsky Associates; our publisher, Will Kiester; our editor, Jill Alexander; and our development editor, Tere Stouffer. Their insight and guidance helped bring clarity and organization to our pages of survey results.

Finally, I must thank my coauthor, Dana Fredsti, a million times over for being willing to join me on this crazy journey, which occasionally resembled a forced march (sorry about that, Dana). I bet she never imagined, back when we were 14-year-olds scribbling away in our rooms, that one day we'd end up asking friends and complete strangers such nosy questions about their sex lives—and writing about it. Thanks for being there, dear friend. This has been more fun than I'd ever have imagined. (And now can we open that nice bottle of wine?)

—**Cynthia W. Gentry**

About the Authors

Dana Fredsti

Dana Fredsti is an ex-B-movie actress with a background in theatrical sword-fighting. Through seven-plus years of volunteering at EFBC/FCC (Exotic Feline Breeding Facility/ Feline Conservation Center), Dana has had a full-grown leopard sit on her feet, been kissed by tigers, held baby jaguars, and had her thumb sucked by an ocelot with nursing issues. She's addicted to bad movies and any book or film, good or bad, that includes zombies. Her other hobbies include surfing (badly), collecting beach glass (obsessively), and wine tasting (happily).

Dana was coproducer/writer/director for a mystery-oriented theatrical troupe based in San Diego. These experiences were the basis for her mystery novel *Murder for Hire: The Peruvian Pigeon*. This book is Dana's second writing partnership with Cynthia Gentry, after *Secret Seductions*, for which Dana used the pseudonym Roxanne Colville.

Dana has written numerous published articles, essays, and shorts, including stories in *Cat Fantastic*, an anthology series edited by Andre Norton; *Danger City*; and *Mondo Zombie*. Her essays can be found in *Morbid Curiosity*, issues 2 through 7. Additionally, she has written and produced several low-budget screenplays and currently has another script under option. Dana was also cowriter/associate producer on *Urban Rescuers*, a documentary on feral cats and TNR (Trap/Neuter/ Return), which won Best Documentary at the 2003 Valley Film Festival in Los Angeles. Under the nom de plume Inara LaVey, she has written several short stories, including *Succubusted*, and two novels, *Ripping the Bodice*, and *Champagne*, out at Ravenous Romance, a new e-book site focused on erotic romance.

Dana is currently working on the second book in the Murder for Hire series, *The Big Snooze*. And Inara is working on her third novel for Ravenous.

Cynthia W. Gentry

Cynthia W. Gentry has written, much to her surprise, several books about sex. She's the coauthor, with her husband, Nima Badiey, of *What Men Really Want in Bed: The Surprising Facts Men Wish Women Knew About Sex*. She also coauthored *Secret Seductions: 62 Naughty Nights, Lusty Liaisons, and Sexy Surprises*, with Roxanne Colville, and is the author of *The Bedside Orgasm Book: 365 Days of Sexual Ecstasy*, reissued in paperback as *Mind-Blowing Orgasms Every Day: 365 Wild and Wicked Ways to Revitalize Your Sex Life*. She wrote the erotica for David Ramsdale's *Red Hot Tantra: Erotic Secrets of Red Tantra for Intimate, Soul-to-Soul Sex and Ecstatic, Enlightened Orgasms*.

She is frequently interviewed by magazines like *Glamour* and *Cosmopolitan* for articles about sex and relationships.

Cynthia's short fiction has appeared in *Area i, The Montserrat Review*, and *Reed Magazine*, and on the e-book site Ravenous Romance, and her nonfiction has been published online and in magazines such as *budget savvy*. Her essay "Following Anaïs: How I Rediscovered My Libido in a Single Night" appeared in the anthology *HerStory: What I Learned in My Bathtub . . . and More True Stories on Life, Love, and Other Inconveniences*. She has covered film festivals for indiWIRE.com and has written for the Literary Arts section of SFStation.com.

Cynthia has a master's degree in journalism from the University of California at Berkeley and a BA in English from Stanford University. She lives in Northern California with her husband and son. Read Cynthia's blog, The Mind Reels, at the-mind-reels.blogspot.com, or visit her website at www.cwgentry.com.

Index

afterglow
  cold shoulder, 134
  communication and, 127–128
  criticism and, 136–137
  cuddling, 126–127, 130
  emotional connection and, 128–129
  enjoyment of, 131
  falling asleep, 129, 130–131
  "hit and run," 136
  hygiene and, 132, 137–138
  mistakes to avoid, 139–141
  passing gas, 140
  past relationships and, 139
  pets and, 138
  rude remarks, 139
  second helpings and, 132
  survey results, 126, 129
anal stimulation
  infection concerns, 46
  intercourse, 108, 115, 156
  oral sex and, 72, 73, 74
  touching, 42, 45, 46, 49, 71

Badiey, Nima, 10, 12
blindfolds, 72, 150, 152, 164
bondage, 107, 115, 163–164
breasts
  areolas, 73
  as erogenous zone, 27, 73
  nipples, 20, 27, 36, 60, 61, 73, 121
  touching, 20, 25, 36, 46, 61, 73

clitoris
  communication and, 52, 61
  foreplay and, 26, 40, 41
  intercourse and, 85, 87, 89, 97, 98
  location of, 60–61
  oral sex and, 62, 64, 69, 70, 71
  orgasms and, 48, 62, 84, 97, 98, 112, 115, 122

  sensitivity of, 20, 36, 44, 60–61, 64, 122
  survey results, 41
  touching, 20, 36, 40, 41, 44, 45, 47, 48
Clooney, George, 115

domination, 107, 115, 163, 165

erogenous zones
  oral sex and, 73–74
  patience and, 19–20, 45
  preferences, 27–28
  touching, 27–28, 44

fantasies
  acting on, 146–147
  bondage and domination, 163–165
  celebrities and, 115, 144, 145
  communication and, 147–149
  erotica, 161–162
  frequency of, 144
  inclusion in, 144, 151, 157, 166, 167
  mistakes to avoid, 156–157
  other women and, 151
  reality and, 146–147, 149
  role-playing, 154–155
  survey results, 147, 153, 155, 158, 159, 162, 163, 167
  threat of, 144–145
  threesomes, 152, 157
  topics of, 150–153, 154–155
  voyeurism, 153
fellatio. See also oral sex.
  aggressiveness and, 76–77
  ejaculation, 79
  enthusiasm for, 75, 77, 78, 79
  feedback on, 78
  head-grabbing, 75–76
  hip-thrusting, 76
  hygiene and, 78–79
  mood and, 77

physical demands of, 79
survey results, 77
Fitzgerald, David, 11
foreplay
   boredom and, 30
   creativity, 20–21
   emotional implications of, 16
   gentleness, 20
   household chores as, 26
   hygiene and, 28, 30
   importance of, 16, 31
   kissing, 24–25
   length of, 16–18
   massage as, 25
   masturbation as, 26
   mental foreplay, 13, 22, 24
   mistakes to avoid, 28, 29, 30
   mood and, 17, 22, 28
   oral sex as, 26, 63
   orgasms and, 16
   past relationships and, 30
   personal enjoyment of, 21
   repetition, 30
   selfishness and, 30
   signals, 18, 21
   survey results, 23, 29
   teasing, 19–20
   touching, 25–26, 28
Fredsti, Dana, 10, 11

Gentry, Cynthia, 10
The Good Vibrations Guide to Sex (Cathy
   Winks/Anne Semans), 17
G-spot
   intercourse and, 97, 98
   location of, 26, 47
   touching, 42, 47, 71

intercourse
   aggressiveness, 107
   bedrooms, 90

clitoral stimulation and, 85, 87, 89, 97, 98
communication and, 84, 85, 94–95, 105,
   108
dirty talk, 95, 107
distractions and, 102, 108, 140
enjoyment of, 82, 84, 85, 86, 107, 108, 113,
   115, 127, 138
enthusiasm for, 82, 109
erectile dysfunction and, 107–108
exotic locations for, 92
fantasies, 101
focus and, 82
frequency, 102–105
G-spot and, 97, 98
honesty and, 105
hotels, 90, 92
hygiene and, 90
intimacy, 83, 85–86, 97, 106
length of, 107
locations for, 90, 91, 92–93
lubrication, 83, 84, 107
missionary position, 96, 97, 99, 100
mistakes to avoid, 106–108
mood and, 99–100
obligation and, 106
orgasms and, 86–87, 97, 98, 108, 112, 113,
   115
outdoors, 90
passing gas and, 140
penis size and, 87–89
phone calls and, 140
physical readiness for, 35
positions, 96–101, 112
pregnancy and, 102
public places and, 92
quickies, 15, 19, 84
rear entry, 98–99, 112
rhythm, 84, 98, 106
second helpings, 132
selfishness and, 106
signals, 82, 95

speed, 83–84, 106
spontaneity and, 100–101
stress and, 102
survey results, 89, 91, 93, 94, 95, 96, 103, 104
touching and, 84, 85, 86, 97, 98, 106
variety, 84, 99–100, 100–101
woman on top, 96, 98, 99, 112

kissing
    afterglow and, 126, 127, 141
    erogenous zones, 27, 73–74
    facial hair and, 186
    as foreplay, 18
    mastering, 24–25
    seduction and, 17, 177
    signals, 176

lubrication, 45, 48, 83, 84, 107

masturbation. See also touching.
    as education, 52, 53
    as foreplay, 26
    observation, 51–53
    participation in, 51–52
    survey results, 51, 53

oral sex. See also fellatio.
    anus and, 72, 73, 74
    blindfolds and, 72
    breasts and, 73
    clitoris and, 62, 64, 69, 70, 71
    communication and, 58, 59, 66, 68
    enthusiasm for, 56, 57–58, 64, 72
    erogenous zones, 73–74
    experimentation, 67
    as foreplay, 26, 63
    hygiene and, 74
    individual preferences, 56–57
    limitations, 74, 75
    as "main event," 57

mistakes to avoid, 64, 65
mood and, 63
orgasms and , 59, 60, 62, 63
perineum and, 73, 74
pressure, 66, 67
reassurance and, 58, 62
rhythm, 62, 66, 67
sensitivity, 59, 60–61
signals, 58, 66, 68
speed, 61–62
survey results, 65, 67, 68, 74, 75
tongue techniques, 69–70
touching and, 48, 60, 61, 70–71
trust and, 57, 72
variety, 61, 72–73
orgasms
    additional stimulation and, 34, 84
    clitoris and, 48, 62, 84, 97, 98, 112, 115, 122
    communication and, 114–115
    complimenting, 52
    difficulty achieving, 112–115, 121, 197–198
    faking, 118, 119, 120–121
    foreplay and, 16
    intercourse and, 86–87, 97, 98, 108, 112, 113, 115
    missionary position and, 97
    multiple orgasms, 122, 123
    oral sex and, 59, 60, 62, 63
    physical reaction to, 121, 122
    position and, 85, 112
    rhythm and, 35, 61, 62, 66
    sensitivity following, 60, 85
    sexual enjoyment and, 86–87, 108, 115
    stress and, 112, 113
    survey results, 112, 114, 116, 118, 119, 121, 123
    techniques, 115, 116, 117
    vagina and, 87, 112, 121
    woman on top position and, 98
oxytocin, 27, 128–129

pornography, 159–162

quickies, 15, 19, 84, 86

seduction
  appearance and, 179, 181, 180, 183
  body hair and, 186
  communication and, 170
  confidence and, 178, 182, 187, 197
  desire and, 171
  emotional stability and, 183, 197
  familiarity and, 170
  favorite body parts, 184, 185, 186–187
  first impressions, 179, 180, 181–183
  hands and, 186–187
  humor and, 182
  initiating, 173–175, 193–196
  intelligence and, 183
  mental seduction, 177–178
  mistakes to avoid, 190
  patience and, 172–173
  romance, 177
  signals, 175, 176, 188
  sincerity, 176–177
  subtlety, 176
  survey results, 179, 180, 185, 189, 191, 195
  timing, 191–192
  touching and, 175
Semans, Anne, 17
SurveyMonkey.com, 12

touching. *See also* masturbation.
  aggressiveness, 44–45, 45–46
  all-over touching, 19, 25, 34, 42, 50, 73
  anticipation and, 35
  anal stimulation, 42, 45, 46, 49, 71
  boundaries and, 39
  breasts, 20, 25, 36, 46, 61, 73
  clitoris, 20, 36, 40, 41, 44, 45, 47, 48
  confidence and, 37

firmness of, 36–37
groping, 44
G-spot, 42, 47, 71
impatience, 44, 45
intercourse and, 84
mistakes to avoid, 44–46
oral sex and, 48, 60, 61, 70–71
personal enjoyment of, 39
rear entry and, 49
seduction and, 175
signals, 38–39, 46
survey results, 41, 43
vagina, 47–48, 49, 62, 71
variety, 34, 37–38
toys, 21, 84, 87, 90, 99, 113, 115, 158

vagina
  orgasms and, 87, 112, 121
  self-consciousness about, 62
  touching, 47–48, 49, 62, 71
  vaginismus, 107
vibrators. *See* toys.

*What Men Really Want in Bed: The Surprising
    Secrets Men Wish Women Knew About
    Sex* (Cynthia Gentry/Nima Badiey),
    10, 11, 21, 31, 51, 55, 98, 109, 114,
    120, 159
Winks, Cathy, 17